Role of Positive … a Moderator of the Occupational Stress-Health Relationship

Shashi Prabha Kashyap

CONTENTS

Preface

Supervisors arewell-rounded employeesin any organization.They serves very pressure-filled job andare willing to accept the responsibilities required to keep an organization running. Butover the past few decades, the nature of work has changed dramatically. The modernization and technological changes in organizations are at a very increasing rate. These changes in organizationsreflect in employee's behavior in various spheres of their lives and workplace as a resultant effect of stress. Stress in employees results from interactions between employees and their environment that are perceived as straining or exceeding their adaptive capacities and threatening their health and well-being. The element of perception indicates that individual stress responses reflect differences in personality as well as differences in their physical strength or general health.

The present study describes a system in which the work environment contains stress for employees because of their personal and health orientation. Those employees were using various coping methods to deal with this stress. The success of this study, in combination with the intensity of the stress as well as a number of personal variables/attributes, interacts to reduce a level of stress and keep good health of the employees. It is expected that results obtained may through light on issue, which though quit important, have escaped the interest and attention of researchers so for. Furthermore, they may also contribute in formulating programs and employee's counselors to provide the necessary support and assistance to supervisors and it is an attempt to explore the employees from other levels of organization was also undertaken.

The thesis consists of seven chapters. The *first* chapter deals with an introduction of the problem along with a brief explanation of concepts and theories related to the psychological aspects concerning the key variables of proposed research such as stress, occupational stress, health, resilience, optimism and positive affectivity.

The *second* chapter includes the review of literature relevant in context to the research variables under study and those which focus on the relationship between these variables. The *third* chapter presents the statement of the problem in the present research, rational of the present study, followed by the objectives and hypotheses.

The *fourth* chapter presents methodology in which the description of sample on which the study was conducted, design of the study utilized in this investigation, tools of measurement, procedure of the data collection and statistical analyses are described. The *fifth* chapter includes the description of the results obtained from the statistical analysis of responses of the subjects on psychometric tools used in the present study and which have been presented in tabular and graphical from.

The *sixth* chapter presents discussion of the results in the light of relevant research literature available in the field. The final *seventh* chapter presents summary and conclusions. This chapter provides a brief resume of the whole research along with recommendations based on the obtained results.

Department of Psychology,
Faculty of Social Sciences,
Banaras Hindu University,
Varanasi-221005, INDIA.
May, 29, 2015

(ShashiPrabhaKashyap)

Chapter-I

INTRODUCTION

Supervisory level employees play an important role in any organization. Supervisors in a production or manufacturing organization typically serve as a member of team leadership and are considered a technical professional within the organization. As such the production supervisor, organization provides difficult technical tasks that is, oversees the planning, scheduling, setup and running of routine or special production streams, manages the dispersal and distribution of materials for production, material labor and material requirements to meet the daily production schedule, oversees the work of production and production support staff, communicates expectations and provides direction and training, monitors work performance and provide feedback, coordinates maintenance of production equipment, etc. So it can be said that supervisors perform a wide range of functions, all of which are closely intertwined. They serves very pressure-filled job. In other words it must be said that supervisors must be well-rounded employees who are willing to accept the responsibilities required to keep an organization running. But it is a matter of concern over the past few decades, the nature of work has changed dramatically by changes in science and technology at work, the globalization in many industries, organizational restructuring, remarkable growth of economy, downsizing, changes in work constructs and work time scheduling have radically transformed the nature of work. In organization these changes reflects in employee's behavior to be experience and feels moderate to high degree of psychological, physiological and social disturbances in various spheres of their lives and workplace as a resultant effect of stress. Consistently increasing rate of high stress leads to deteriorate physical as well as psychological health of employees.

Employee effective job performance depends upon their cognitive ability to deal with workplace demands. However, while some employees are severely damaged under situations of heavy stress, others are not; i.e. the stressful situation does not always have absolute or unconditional association with adverse outcomes. The stress-strain model, therefore, hypothesized existence of moderators that can moderate the impact of stress on strain. These moderators include internal characteristics (i.e. personal attributes), and situational characteristics or psychological variables such as, coping style, self-efficacy, emotional stability, hope, happiness, hardiness, optimism, emotional intelligence, resilience and positive affectivity that affects employee's attitudes toward work. Among these variables resilience, optimism and positive affectivity emerge as a boosters for the employee's in this investigation.

This study describes a system in which the work environment contains stress for employees because of their personal and health orientation. Those employees were using various coping methods to deal with this stress. The success of this study, in combination with the intensity of the stress as well as a number of personal variables/attributes, interacts to reduce a level of stress and keep good health of the employees.

STRESS

Every living thing on the earth encounters stress in one degree or another. One in five people suffer from stress, with half a million people reporting they have become ill due to stress. Right from the time of birth till death, an individual is invariably exposed to various stressful situations. In fact, modern times have been called the "age of anxiety and stress" (Coleman, 1976). So stress has become an integral part of everyday living. Stress can arise from any situation or thought that makes you tense; feel frustrated, angry, nervous or anxious. Stress is not necessarily bad in small doses, it can help people perform under pressure and motivate them to do their best. But, beyond a certain point, stress stops being helpful and starts causing damage to health, mood, productivity, relationships, and quality of life. With so many factors and events that can contribute to stress. It can be difficult to define the concept of "stress." Selye coined the word "stress". The term stress has been derived from the Latin word "stringere" which means 'to draw tight.' It has been used in the English language since about fifteenth century, when it had the meaning of pressure or physical strain. Various terms are synonymously used with stress viz. anxiety, frustration, conflict, pressure, hardship, strain, adversity or affliction, etc.

On the basis for our knowledge of the concept of stress was laid more than a century ago by the French scientist Claude Bernard. He was the first to recognize how the body endeavors to maintain a relatively constant internal state in an ever-changing environment (Bernard, 1878). A few decades later, the stress reaction was described by Walter Cannon (1929) and Hans Selye (1936) as actions taken by the body in situations where the internal homeostasis is threatened. Selye (1936) discovered that a range of stimuli of varying nature increased blood levels of cortisol by provoking activation of the hypothalamic-pituitary-adrenal (HPA) axis. He called this phenomenon the "general adaptation syndrome" (GAS). The GAS has three stages, i.e., alarm, resistance, and collapse. The alarm stage is the body's initial response to stressor, e.g., increase heart rate and blood pressure, and release of glucose to provide energy for action. If the stress is prolonged, the stage of resistance emerges. The process of homeostasis comes into play at this stage; the body tries to maintain equilibrium. There is continuing effort to adapt to the stressor during this stage; the body cannot go on coping with stress indefinitely. The third stage of collapse is characterized by a loss of resistance to the stressor, and exhaustion, collapse and even death can occur. But this has been challenged by the stress researchers as it does not give any significance to cognitive processes and individual differences in these physical responses to stressors.

Lazarus (1966) argued that stress is unique to each individual and dependent on appraisal (perception of stress). Lazarus believed that an individual appraises a situation and if it is stressful, the person starts using coping skills. The person makes the best response possible and actively defines and shapes stressful transactions by means of his cognitive appraisals and coping responses (David & Suls, 1999; DeLongis & Holtzman, 2005). According to some researchers the experience of stress can alter the way a person feels thinks and behaves; and can also produce changes in their physiological functions (Stansfeld, Fuhrer, Shipley, & Marmot, 1999; Sauter & Murphy, 1995). Selye (1980) stated that "the concept of stress is still fraught with definitional contradictions, and suffers from the mixed blessing of being too well known and too little understood."

The term stress denotes different things to so many different people that it has been described as the most imprecise in the scientific dictionary. There are literally hundreds of definitions for stress to be found in the research and professional literatures. However, the concept of stress seems to had a special place in the mind of laymen and scientists ever since Selye (1956) defined stress as "non-specific responses of the body to any demand made upon it," his opinion was that organism makes a universal pattern to response to all types of internal or external demands made on the body. The mental and physical condition that results from a perceived threat or demand that cannot be dealt with readily and our response to events that disrupt, or threaten to disrupt our physical or psychological functioning (Lazarus & Folkman, 1984; Taylor, 1999), the rate of all the wear and tear caused by life (Selye, 1956), the body's reaction to a change that requires a physical, mental or emotional adjustment or response (Medical definition). The term stress has been used to refer to the response to stressors (Beehr & Franz 1987; Caplan, Cobb & French, 1975; Caplan, Cobb, French, Harrison & Pinneau, 1975; Kahn & Quin, 1970).

Stress can also refer to the subjective perception of events as threatening or negative, the idea being that the impact of stress depends upon how an individual appraises that event (Baum, Cohen, & Hall, 1993). So stress is regarded as predominantly subjective in nature, rather than an objective phenomenon. It is "a process in which environmental demands that tax or exceed the adaptive capacity of the organism, resulting in psychological and biological changes which place the person at risk for disease." (Cohen, Kessler, & Gordon, 1995). It is a psychological perturbation from homeostasis, such as hormonal changes, disturbed sleep, fatigue, and infertility that indicate effects of a stressor on an organism (Greil, 1997; Kales, Soldatos, & Kales, 1987; Maier & Watkin, 1998; Selye, 1955).

According to Srivastava, (1999) psychological stress is not a simple event, but is a process which comprises following successive events:

1. Perception of some unusual, demanding noxious or adverse situation or event.
2. Cognitive appraisal by the focal person of the demands or threats, and probably undesirable consequence of the situation, and of his capabilities and available resources.
3. Emergence of a state of emotional disequilibrium spontaneously followed by deviant or unhealthy psychological, physiological and biochemical responses.
4. Operation of adaptive or coping efforts by the focal person at cognitive and behavioral levels.

Stress therefore, may be referred to as a, "deviant psycho-physiological state of the individual resulting from a situation cognitively appraised as excessively demanding or threatening, and requiring the focal person to make some adaptive efforts to cope with it" (Srivastava, 1999). "Stress may be defined as a threat, real or implied, to the psychological or physiological integrity of an individual" (McEwen, 1999). European Agency for Safety and healthy at work (2000) defined stress as a, "psychological state which is part of and reflects a wider process of interaction between the person and their work environment." Krumm (2007) viewed that stress is the term pertains to the response of people to the demands placed on them. This includes many of the normal pressure most people experience at work. For example, a person's preparation for work could be measured as more stressful than resting in bed, but preparation for work is usually considered necessary and beneficial. According to Schultz (2002) stress is the combination of physiological and psychological responses to excessive and usually unpleasant stimulation and to threatening events in the environment. Lovallo (2005) defines Stress as an environmental demand that can if too intense or prolonged disrupt healthy functioning.

Stress show itself in a number of ways. For instance, an individual who is experiencing a high level of stress may develop high blood pressure, ulcers, irritability, difficult in making routine decisions, loss of appetite and accident proneness (Sabatino et al., 2004). The term stress is sometimes used to refer external environmental stimuli or demands that tax on organism's systems. These demands, or stressors, can vary in number, duration, and severity, and can be evoked within the laboratory or occur within the natural environment (Segerstrom & Miller, 2004). Similarly, Gerigg and Zimbardo (2005) defined it as a partner of reposes an organism makes to stimulus events that disturb the equilibrium and tax or exceed its ability to cope. The individual's response to, or evaluation of stressful events also has an important role to play. Researchers have typically referred to this response/evaluation as stress. Stress is an internal event that is subjectively defined. Matteson and Ivancevich (1987) have believe stress is a consequence of any action, situation or event that places demands on a person (i.e., stress is a consequence of stressors), that is both an adaptive response and moderated by individual differences.

The most commonly definition of stress may be categorized into three types. The first type is stimulus-based which considers stress as a situational or environmental-based stimulus, impinging on the person. The second type is response-based, defining stress as an individual's psychological or physiological response to environmental/situational forces. The third definition, applies an interactive approach often called the stressor-strain approach. All of them can be placed into one of the two categories i.e. stress as a stimulus (source of stress or stressor) and stress as a response (outcome or manifestation of stress or strain). In other words, stress can be seen as a force acting on a person and causing discomfort. It is an emotional, mental or physical strain in response to a stressor (event, person, situation, and thing). In general, we can say that stress is related to both external and internal factors. Stress refers to external pressure that is exerted on a person, which in turn results in tension or "strain" (Kahn & Byosiere, 1992). External factors include the physical environment, including your job, your relationship with others, your home and all the situations, challenges, difficulties and expectations you're confronted with a daily basis. Internal factors which influence the ability to handle stress include nutritional states, overall health and fitness levels, emotional well-being and the amount of sleep and rest we get.

OCCUPATIONAL STRESS:

Occupational stress is a growing concern for employees and employers not only in India but all over the world. The structure of the organization itself can also be a source of stress for employees. For example, hierarchical, top-down management structures that provide workers with little or no say in the decision-making process, restrictions on behavior, office politics, lack of effective consultation, and erratic working hours can all have detrimental effects on workers' health or well-being. Occupational stress, job stress, and work stress are common terms in the area's literature that have overlapping meaning. The researchers in the area of organizational psychology and management have used the term job stress/occupational stress to denote employee's mental state aroused by a job situation or a combination of job situations perceived as presenting excessive and divergent demands.

Stress at work place has become an integral part of everyday life and is referred as 'worldwide epidemic 'by the World Health Organization. In 1994/95 only 17% of stress claims were made for workplace trauma, aggression and assault with the remainder being based on more pervasive and chronic causes, including interpersonal conflicts, and organizational factors such as change and pressure to meet deadlines. It is not surprising, therefore, that the search for causes of organizational strain and its link with other important outcome variables such as job satisfaction. Stress is often developed when an individual is assigned a major responsibility without proper authority and delegation of power. Stress also develops when an individual feels he is not competent to undertake the role assigned to him effectively. The individual feels that he or she lacks knowledge, skill and training on performing the role.

Beer and Newman (1978) defines occupational stress as "A condition arising from the interaction of people and their jobs and characterized by changes within people that force them to deviate from their normal functioning" identified thirty seven job or organizational characteristics that might be occupational stressors and these were split in to four categories: job demands and task characteristics, role demands or expectations, organizational characteristics or conditions, organization's external demands and conditions. Caplan, Cobb and French (1975) have accordingly defined occupational stress as "any characteristics of job environment which poses a threat to the individual." Health and Safety Executive defined occupational stress as "The adverse reaction people have to excessive pressures or other types of demand placed on them."

Stress is a common feature of organization life, across all occupation domains (Cooper, 1998; Hancock & Desmond, 2001). But some other stress researchers have tried to define it in terms of interaction between worker and work environment. The stress fullness of a job situation or a factor is determined not only by the divergent or threatening demands of the situation but by how the individual perceive and evaluates it with reference to his own capability and characteristics. Stress denotes the psychological state experienced by an employee when faced with demands, constraints, and or opportunities that have important but uncertain outcomes (Bheer & Bhagat, 1985; Schuler, 1980). NIOSH (2004) defines job stress as the harmful physical and emotional responses that occur when the requirements of the job do not match the capabilities, resources, or needs of the workers.

Stress has been identified as one of the key problems in the workforce for the next century (Keichel, 1993). Annually in absenteeism, lost productivity, accidents and medical insurance (Laws, 1996). Various studies have revealed that workers suffering from stress exhibit decreased productivity, absenteeism, higher number accidents, lower morale and greater interpersonal conflict with colleagues and superiors (Cranwell and Alyssa, 2005). Stress in the workplace can affect communication effectiveness, the ability to focus on job and decision making ability. A huge and multi field's literature points a lot of key factors such as work environment, management support, workload etc. Workplace stress is attributed to role ambiguity (Beer, 1995), and interpersonal conflicts (Narayanan, Menon, & Spector, 1999). Stress causes absenteeism and can lead to other problems such as drug addiction, alcoholism, depression, and poor job performance.

Survey of the literature on occupational stress reveals that there are a number of factors related to job which affect the behavior of the employees and as a result of it, normal life is disturbed (McLean, 1974; Brief, Schular and Vansell, 1981) and this kind of stress related effects of work are one of the most costly problems for many organizations. Current estimates in the United States of the cost of stress in workplace range from $200 billion to $300 billion annually (Farren, 1999). Those costs include absenteeism; diminished productivity, employee turnover, accidents, directs medical, legal, and insurance fees; and workers compensation awards (Arsenault & Dolan, 1983; Siu, 2002). In 1990, the United States' National Institute of Occupational Safety and Health (NIOSH) declared occupational stress to be one of the 10 leading causes of workplace death (Sauter, Murphy, & Hurrell, 1990) and it is now common to speak of occupational stress as an epidemic (Quick, Quick, Nelson, & Hurrell, 1997).

It has been observed that in psychology there has been little empirical research examining multiple stressors (Evans, Allen, Tafalla, & O'Meara 1996). While some research has been directed towards overcoming this problem, it remains the case that few studies are conducted that look at other contextual factors. There are a number of elements within the work environment that can be classified as stressors. Factors that are intrinsic to the job include poor working conditions, work overload and under load, time pressures, physical danger, and shift work (Cooper & Cartwright, 1994). According to Vakola & Nikolaou (2005) different stressors in work can be categorized to be caused by content, working conditions, employment conditions and social relations at work.

Some stress researchers have emphasized the role of job situations in their definition of job or occupational stress. Sources of stress pertaining to the employee's role in the organization include responsibility for lives, role ambiguity, and role conflict (Sutherland & Cooper, 2000). Role stress has been widely recognized as an antecedent of occupational stress of the many job condition factors proposed as sources of stress at work (Cooper & Marshall, 1976, House & Rizzo, 1972, Miles & Perreault, 1976). Kahn, Wolfe, Quinn, Snoek and Rosenthal (1964) proposed that role stress comprised of three kinds of stresses: role conflict, role ambiguity and role overload. Role conflict is defined as the simultaneous occurrence of two or more sets of pressures in the way that compliance with the one makes it difficult to comply with the other (Orpen, 1982). Role ambiguity is defined in terms of the lack of clarity of role expectations and demands and lack of predictability of behavioral outcomes (Martin, 1992). Role overload is defined as a condition in which an individual is assigned more work than he or she can effectively handle (Miles & Perreault, 1976).

Srivastava & Singh (1984) defines twelve dimensions of occupational stress like;

I. Role overload: It covers job situations like workload, staff insufficiency, lack of time, personal problems, job dissatisfaction, etc.
II. Role ambiguity: It is characterized by vague and insufficient information related to job role; vague and poor planning of job, and vague expectations by colleagues and supervisors, etc.

III. Role conflict: Contradictory instructions from higher officers, interference of officials into the working conditions, vague instructions and insufficient facilities regarding new assignments, contradiction between office instructions and formal working procedures., difficulty in implementing new procedures and policies, etc., are included in this dimension.

IV. Unreasonable group and political pressures: This dimension covers the difficulty to adjust with the political and group pressures and formal rules and instructions, compulsion to perform unwillingly, maintenance of group conformity, violation of formal procedures and policies, etc.

V. Responsibility for person: This dimension covers such aspects as the thrust of responsibility of other persons, the responsibility of other employees, future, responsibility for progress of organization, etc.

VI. Under-participation: This dimension covers job areas such as the position of the person in the organization that with high or low power the acceptance of suggestions made by other persons, etc.

VII. Powerlessness: This dimension covers areas such as acceptance of decisions taken by the person among employees, acceptance of suggestions regarding training programs of employees, lack of coordination of interest and opinion in making appointments for important posts, etc.

VIII. Poor peer relationships: The area covered under this dimension refers to poor interpersonal relationships with colleagues, colleagues' attempt to defame and malign the employee as unsuccessful, colleagues' lack of cooperation in solving administrative and industrial problems, lack of cooperation and team spirit of employees of the organization, etc.

IX. Intrinsic impoverishment: monotonous nature of assignment, opportunity, to utilize abilities and experience independently, opportunity to develop aptitude and proficiency, place of suggestion in problem solving, etc., are included in this area.

X. Low status: This dimension covers respect received by an employee from others, the role of nature of the job in enhancing social status, due significance given by higher authorities to the post and work, etc.

XI. Strenuous working conditions: This dimension covers tense circumstances in which work has to be done, risky and complicated assignments, unsatisfactory working conditions from the point of view of welfare and convenience, etc.

XII. Unprofitability: Low salary, absence of rewards, lack of motivation, etc., are included here.

Other sources of stress may come from relationships with co-workers or management, dissatisfaction with career development opportunities, and a lack of job security (Parker & DeCotiis, 1983). According to Kumar (2006), there are six sources of stressful situations have been suggested which may affect the human behavior in industrial setting, namely:

1. Task based stress (difficulty, ambiguity, work load etc.)

2. Role based stress (conflict, ambiguity, role etc.)

3. Stress intrinsic to the behavior setting (e.g., effects of crowding under manning, etc.)

4. Stress arising from the physical environment itself (e.g. extreme cold hostile forces, etc.)

5. Stress arising from the social environment, in the sense of inter-personal relations, (e.g., interpersonal disagreement, privacy, and isolation, etc.)

6. Stress within the person system, which the focal person 'brings with him' to the situation (e.g., anxiety, perceptual style, etc.)

According to Harrington (2013), there are a number of theoretical models of organizational stress, but five of the most popular are the organizational role stress, the person-environment fit, the job demands-control, the effort-reward imbalance (ERI), and he organizational injustice model. A brief survey of each model as follows:

ORGANIZATIONAL ROLE STRESS MODEL:

The outlined in their book entitled organizational stress: Studies in role conflict and Ambiguity, Robert Kahn and his associates (Kahn, Wolfe, Quinn, Snoek, & Rosenthal, 1964) established organizational role theory as one of the first major theoretical frameworks specific to the scientific study of stress in the workplace. In their view, stress involves adjustment to work roles. A work role was described by Beehr and Glazer (2005, p.10), "work role can be defined as the social character one plays in an organization." Although there are many elements to Kahn and his colleagues (1964) model of organizational role stress known as the role episode model, the most widely studied concepts from their model are role conflict, role ambiguity, and role overload. According to this model:

Role Conflict: Two or more role demands are incompatible with each other. For example, being a responsible worker means working overtime to complete your work tasks, but being a responsible parent means going to your child's soccer game instead. This role conflict creates stress.

Role Ambiguity: The duties, responsibilities, and performance expectations of the job are not clearly defined by organizational leaders. For example, a new worker in an organization is unsure how much time to devote to report writing and how much to spend improving sagging customer relations. As a result, the new employee experiences stress.

Role overload: The work load is too great and there are insufficient resources to complete the tasks assigned in the time provided, an experience referred to as quantitative overload, or the employee does not have the required competencies to complete the tasks even when there is sufficient time, an experience known as qualitative overload.

PERSON-ENVIRONMENT FIT MODEL:

Another model of organizational stress, the person-environment (P-E) fit model (Edwards, Caplan, & Harrison, 1998), states that stress occurs when there is a poor fit between the worker and the work environment. Determination of a misfit is subjective and occurs when a worker perceives that his or her

1. Abilities do not match the demands of the organization or

2. Needs are not met by the organization - the greater the misfit, the greater the stress. For example, an elementary school teacher who enjoys working with young children is a better fit than one who feels more comfortable working with adults. All things being equal, the teacher who prefers working with children would experience less P-E fit stress than the one who prefers working with adults.

JOB DEMANDS-CONTROL (JOB-STRAIN) MODEL:

In the job demands-control (also known as job-strain) model (Karasek, 1979), strain occurs when a worker experiences high psychological job demands yet has little control over the job. This lack of control is known as low decision latitude, a condition characterized by having insufficient skills or authority over one's job to complete the job tasks autonomously. For example, according to this model, which medical professionals should have more strain, nurses or physicians? If we guessed nurses then we are correct. Because nurses have high psychological demands combined with low decision latitude (low control) (Brown, James, & Mills, 2006) because they have less patient care decision-making authority than physicians. Physicians provide the patient care directives and nurses follow them rather than the other way around.

EFFORT-REWARD IMBALANCE (ERI) MODEL:

The effort-reward imbalance (ERI) model (Siegrist, 1996) Proposes that high-cost, low-gain work efforts are stressful. When we give a lot to our work we expect reciprocity in the way of high reward. The reward pay is in the form of money, status, or esteem. However, when we experience an imbalance in reciprocity, where high work effort is met with low reward we experience distress. This loss of control threatens our sense of mastery and self-efficacy over our occupational role status, resulting in further stress such as fear of being laid off or being passed over for promotion.

ORGANIZATIONAL INJUSTICE MODEL:

The organizational injustice model assumes that stress occurs when the organization interpersonal transactions, procedures, or outcomes are perceived as unfair (Cropanzano, Goldman, & Nenson, 2005). According to this model organizational injustice can occur under a variety of circumstances. For example, organizational injustice occurs when employees are not treated with respect and dignity, if workplace procedures are unethical or inconsistent, or when the organization rewards its employees in ways that are not in proportion to their effort. Therefore, these outcomes are seen as not only unfair but also sources of stress.

According to researcher job stress/occupational stress can lead to poor health and even injury. Long-term exposure to job stress has been linked to an increased risk of musculo-skeletal disorders, depression, and job burnout, and may contribute to a range of debilitating diseases, ranging from cardiovascular disease to cancer.

HEALTH

Health is considered as wealth. In present times people have become more cautious about their health. Health is conceived as positive state of physical, mental and social well-being besides the absence of disease/illness. In health literature it is defined as various ways; Health is a state of complete physical, mental and social well-being and not merely the absence of disease and the good life (Tinetti & Fried, 2004). Most practitioners identified health as the interrelatedness of several factors, physical, mental and spiritual factors. They emphasized health as good functioning, absence of disease and chronic disease (Julliard, Klimenko, & Jacob, 2006).

Health can be divided into two spheres: physical and mental/ psychological. Physical health is the overall condition of living organisms at a given time, the soundness of the body, freedom from disease or abnormality, and the condition of optimal well-being. The main concern in health is preventing injury and healing damage caused by injuries and biological attacks. (Ron Kurtus, 2002). Mental health is undoubtedly an indispensable foundation of human personality used. Mental health is a term to describe either a level of cognitive or emotional well-being or an absence of a mental disorder. During last two decades, mental health has come to be defined in terms of psychological well-being. Low psychological well-being is illustrated in anxiety, depression, low morale, lack of self-confidence, low sense of personal autonomy, inability to cope with the problems of living and dissatisfaction with oneself and the social and physical environment.

Mental health is a state of well-being in which the individual realizes mental health is a state of well-being in which the individual realizes his or her own abilities, can cope with the normal stresses of life, can work productively and fruitfully, and is able to make a contribution to his or her community. Merriam Webster (2009), defined mental health as "a state of psychological well-being in which an individual is able to use his or her cognitive and emotional capabilities, functions in society, and everyday life." Mental health is the capacity to think rationally and logically, and to cope with the transitions, stresses, traumas, and losses that occur in all lives in way that allow emotional stability and growth (Hales & Hales, 1995). People's his or her own abilities, can cope with the normal stresses of life, can work productively and fruitfully, and is able to make a contribution to his or her community (WHO, 1998).

The concept of mental health include subjective well-being, perceived self-efficiency, autonomy, competence, intergenerational dependence and self-actualization of one's intellectual and emotional potential. Mental health is a term used to describe either a level of cognitive or emotional well-being or an absence of a mental disorder (About.com, 2006). In classical Indian tradition, health is considered as a state of delight or a feeling of physical, mental and spiritual wellbeing (Dalal, 2005; Sinha, 1990; Verma, 1998). This Indian perspective is closer to the WHO definition of health; provides an ideal state of human functioning and conceptualizes health as a state of mind which is peaceful, serene, and free from conflicts and desires.

Today positive psychologist's like Ryff and Keyes (1995) have defined complete mental health as the combination of emotional wellbeing, social wellbeing and psychological wellbeing as well as absence of recent mental illness. Emotional wellbeing is presence of positive affect, satisfaction with life and absence of negative affect. Social wellbeing incorporates acceptance, actualization, contribution, coherence and integration and psychological wellbeing combines self-acceptance, personal growth, and purpose in life, environmental mastery, autonomy and positive relationship with others. Mental health generally refers to an individual's thoughts, feelings, and actions particularly when faced with life's challenges and stresses. Good mental health is not just the absence of mental health problems. But it refers to the full and harmonious functioning of the total personality which gives satisfaction and sense of fulfillment.

In general, we can say that health refers how effectively and successfully a person functions, feels is capable and competent, and able to handle normal levels of stress, maintains satisfying relationships and leads an independent life, and is able to "become back" or recover from difficult situations.

RESILIENCE

Etymologically, the word 'resilience' derived from the Latin word 'selire' (to spring) and 'resilier' (spring back). Emmy Werner (1982) was one of the early scientists to use the term resilience in the 1970s and the concept of resilience was first used by child psychiatrist Michel Rutter in his frequently cited article "Resilience in the Face of Adversity", published in 1985. Resilience is the ability to successfully cope with change or misfortune. Resilient individuals regain their balance and keep going, despite adversity and misfortune. They find meaning amidst confusion and tumult. Resilient persons are self-confident and understand their own strengths and abilities. They do not feel a pressure to conform but take pleasure in being unique and will 'go it alone' if necessary. Resilient individuals have confidence in their ability to persevere because they have done so before and anticipate rather than fear change and challenges. Being resilient does not mean that an individual will 'bounce back' and return to the same position after experiencing difficulties, but it does mean that equilibrium will be re-established. Resilient persons experience the same difficulties and stressors as everyone else; they are not immune or hardened to stress, but they have learned how to deal with life's inevitable difficulties and this ability sets them apart.

Masten and colleagues (1990) have identified three different types of resilient phenomena: (1) resilience as overcoming the odds, (2) resilience as stress-resistance, and (3) resilience as recovery. Resilience as overcoming the odds refers to successful adaptation despite the odds against such adaptation. In this process, individuals have been identified as having some type of risk factor (e.g. SES) that would typically predict maladaptation, but they have been able to achieve better-than-expected outcomes despite that risk factor (Luthar et al., 2000). Resilience as stress-resistance implies the process where individuals are faced with acute or chronic stressors but are able to effectively maintain equilibrium under short-term significant strain. Finally, resilience as recovery occurs when individuals are exposed to prolonged or severe threat, and show a decrease in functioning, but are able to recover quicker than most when the threat is no longer present. Resilience is the positive capacity of people to cope with stress. George Vaillant (1993) defines resilience as the "self-righting tendencies" of the person, "both the capacity to be bent without breaking and the capacity, once bent, to spring back". (Goldstein, 1997) Resilience is the capacity to maintain competent functioning in the face of major life stressors.

Kaplan, Turner, Norman and Stillson, (1996) defines resilience as a dynamic process that individuals exhibit positive behavioral adaptation when they encounter significant adversity, trauma, tragedy, threats, or even significant sources of stress. According to Luthar, Cicchetti and Becker, (2000) resilience means the skills, abilities, knowledge, and insight that accumulate over time as people struggle to surmount adversity and meet challenges. The term resilience reflects the ability of individuals to maintain relatively stable mental function throughout the course of events (Bonanno, 2004). It is an ongoing and developing fund of energy and skill that can be used in current struggles. (Garmezy et al., 1994; Saleebey, 1996) Resilience is the capacity for successful adaptation, positive functioning or competence despite high-risk status, chronic stress, or following prolonged or severe trauma. (Egeland, Carlson, & Sroufe, 1993; Sonn & Fisher, 1998) "The outcome from negotiations between individuals and their environments for the resources to define themselves as healthy amidst conditions collectively viewed as adverse" (Ungar, 2004). Resilience is the process by which individuals exhibit successful adaptation despite experiencing adversity (Masten, Best & Garmezy, 1990). Current conceptualizations do not imply that resilience is absolute or unchanging, but instead argue that resilience as a dynamic process of positive adaptation where new strengths emerge as life circumstances change (Luthar et al., 2000).

Resilience is defined primarily in terms of protective factors that resist the life stresses (Kaplan et al., 1996). Resilience is also defined as successful adaptation in response to adversity (Zautra, Hall, & Murray, 2010), In other words we can say that resilience is the ability to roll with the punches. It means that although you encounter stress, adversity, trauma or tragedy, you keep functioning, both psychologically and physically. Resilience is a psychological phenomenon as it is a perception of inner strength that allows for the physical manifestation of that strength, i.e., the quick recovery from disruptions in functioning and return to previous level of functioning (Carver, 1998; Steinhardt & Dolbier, 2008). Resilience is described as value laden in the sense that there is an arbitrary judgment involved in defining of risk factors and adversity. It is sometimes defined as a psychological process developed in response to intense life stressors that facilitate healthy functioning (Johnson et al., 2009). Alternatively, other researchers have described resilience as having three primary components: resilient qualities, the resiliency process and innate resilience. Resilient qualities measure the psychosocial qualities of resilient individuals. The resiliency process describes how the individual adapts to the traumatic event, and innate resilience consists of the identification of motivational factors that may influence the individual's response (Richardson, 2002). Resilience has been defined as the capacity to withstand, regulate and cope with ongoing life challenges and succeeds in maintaining equilibrium despite negative effects from stress (DiCorcia & Tronick, 2011; Montpetit, Bergeman, Deboeck, Tiberio, & Boker, 2010; Neill & Dias, 2001; Schetter & Dolbier, 2011). Resilience emphasizes the ability to recover quickly from disruptions in functioning (Shin, Taylor & Seo, 2012). In an organisational context, Luthans (2002) defines resilience as 'the developable capacity to rebound or bounce back from adversity, conflict, and failure or even positive events, progress, and increased responsibility'.

Resilience is an interactive phenomenon that is inferred from findings indicating that some individuals have a relatively good outcome despite having experienced serious stresses or adversities – their outcome being better than that of other individuals who suffered the same experiences (Rutter, 2013). Although there is still considerable debate regarding definitions of resilience, trait orientation suggests that resilience is a personality trait that helps individuals cope with adversity and achieve good adjustment and development (Hu, Zhang, & Wang, 2015).

Theoretical writings indicate that psychological resilience is a relatively stable personality trait characterized by the ability to overcome, steer through, and bounce back from adversity (Block & Kremen, 1996; Block & Block, 1980). Resilience, which is one of those traits, is defined as the ability to 'rebound' and regain original shape following trauma or shock (Oxford 1989); and the promotion of positive adaptation under stress and adversity (Wagnild 2003). Tugade and Fredrickson (2004) stated that psychological resilience refers to effective coping and adaptation although faced with loss, hardship, or adversity. Carle and Chassin (2004) reported that individuals with high levels of self-reported resilience are particularly likely to use positive emotions to ''bounce back'' from adverse experiences. An increasing number of researchers are also using the concept of resilience to explore how people cope with 'negative life events' and even how individuals negotiate the more ordinary upheavals associated with normal 'life transitions'. Coping with painful events and unpleasant emotions is a struggle for every human being. Those who are less resilient may turn to unhealthy actions or negative beliefs about themselves to cope with the difficulties encountered in their lives (Smokowski, 1999). It is adaptive coping in the face of multiple risk factors (Waller et al., 2003). The various components of resilience can also be thought of having a "buffering" effect between risk factors and negative life outcomes. A research study (Aguirre, 2007; American Psychological Association, 2006; Bonanno, 2004) has shown that resilience is ordinary, not extraordinary, and that people regularly demonstrate being resilient, like;

- Resilience is not a trait that people either have or do not have.
- Resilience involves behaviors, thoughts, and actions that can be learned and developed in anyone.
- Resilience is tremendously influenced by a person's environment.

Research on resilience focuses on those individuals who have overcome difficult life circumstances and have become successful, as well as what factors promote such adaptive functioning.

The traditional approach to resilience is usually centered either on internal qualities such as personality traits, behavioral competence and coping skills (Bartley, Schoon, Mitchell, & Blane, 2010) or only on external social factors such as social and psychological characteristics (Neill & Dias, 2001). Muller (2009) challenged these schools of thoughts by introducing the psychosocial interactive model of resilience, where both the internal and external domains of the individual are considered in the response to stressful conditions. This model takes into account the development over the lifespan where time is a factor for resilience. It is a dynamic process and it can be learned (Neill & Dias, 2001; Rutter, 2012; Spangler et al., 2012). As supported in many research on childhood resilience (Wagnild & Young, 1993) resilience growth may not be in a linear fashion as it can change and develop over time-built or lost-depending on the availabilityof the resilience resources (Muller, 2009; Schetter & Dolbier, 2011).

Similarly, DiCorcia and Tronick (2011) discussed resilience as "a process of regulating everyday life stressors" and that individual of all backgrounds experience stressors in different ways and moderations. This idea is somewhat similar to the transactional model of stress and coping (Lazarus & Folkman, 1984) whereby the regulation of stressors varies according to individual. The Everyday Stress Resilience Hypothesis (DiCorcia & Tronick, 2011) states that resilience growth is dependent on the regulatory success or failure of everyday stress in an individual; the more experience and success in stress regulation, the more equipped an individual is to face greater challenges. DiCorcia and Tronick (2011) presented a well thought of analogy for the Hypothesis: Marathon runners do not run the full marathon distances for stamina training; instead they run a gradual increase of distances in each training over a period of time. The rationale behind the analogy is progressive training develops the runner's stamina. The gradual increase incapacity helps the different muscular and metabolic mechanisms to be prepared for the full distance. Analogous to resilience growth, successfully overcoming adversity or stress builds resilience and prepares one for future stress. However, maintenance training is required to prevent stamina loss, this takes into account the possibilities of resilience being built or lost. Even though DiCorcia and

Tronick (2011) main focus was on infant experiences in stress regulation and resilience growth, their core argument on the Everyday Stress Resilience Hypothesis is applicable to most individuals. Nevertheless, as noted in their review, further research and empirical evidence are needed for the Hypothesis to be valid, in particular, a detailed understanding of individual experiences in self-regulation capacities.

As a response to inconsistencies in understanding resilience, Polk (1997) conducted a meta-analysis that examined 26 research papers to identify the various characteristics and themes that define resilience. She identified four patterns of resilience: dispositional pattern, which encompasses physical and ego-related psychosocial attributes; relational pattern, which refers to the intrinsic and extrinsic characteristics of roles and relationships influencing resilience; situational pattern, which portrays resilience as a capacity for action and assessment in a stressful situation; and the philosophical pattern, which includes personal positive beliefs and reflection. Polk (1997) posited that individuals experience adversity as a force to change.

In summary, to demonstrate resilience, individuals must first encounter adversity and successfully cope and adapt in a positive manner in order to develop resilience to future stress (DiCorcia & Tronick, 2011; Polk, 1997).

According to researcher resilience is the ability to bounce back, take on difficult challenges and still find meaning in life, respond positively to difficult situations, rise above adversity, cope when things look bleak, tap into hope, transform unfavorable situations into wisdom, insight, and compassion. Resilience refers to the ability of an individual, family, organization, or community to cope with adversity and adapt to challenges or change. It is an ongoing process that requires time and effort and engages people in taking a number of steps to enhance their response to adverse circumstances. Resilience implies that after an event, a person or community may not only be able to cope and recover, but also change to reflect different priorities arising from the experience and prepare for the next stressful situation. Resilience is the most important defense people have against stress. It is important to build and foster resilience to be ready for future challenges. Resilience changes over time. It fluctuates depending on how much a person nurtures internal resources or coping strategies. Some people are more resilient in work life, while others exhibit more resilience in their personal relationships. People can build resilience and promote the foundations of resilience in any aspect of life they choose.

POSITIVE AFFECTIVITY

Affect refers to subjective moods and feelings. It was operationalized as the individual's experience of general positive feelings that enhance adaptation. Positive affectivity can be brief, longer lasting, or more stable trait like feelings. Although some use the terms affect, mood, and emotion to distinguish duration, these uses are not applied consistently in the literature, and thus we use these terms interchangeably. Positive Affectivity (PA) reflects the extent to which a person feels enthusiastic, active, and alert. It is described as a person's tendency to be cheerful and energetic, and who experience positive moods (such as pleasure or well-being), across a variety of situations. Individuals who have low levels of positive affectivity tend to be low energy and sluggish or melancholy. High level of positive affectivity represents the extent to which an individual feels energetic and excited, while low level of positive affectivity represents the extent to which an individual feels sadness, sluggishness or weariness (Barsade & Gibson, 2007). Individual high in PA view the world more positive light and report leading full and interesting lives (Watson & Pennebaker, 1989). PA is also strongly related to life satisfaction. PA is associated with positive problem solving approaches (Elliott, Sherwin, Harkins,

& Marmaroush, 1995).The high energy and engagement, optimism, and social interest characteristic of high-PA individuals suggest that they should be more likely to be satisfied with their life. Watson and his colleagues (Watson, 1988; Watson & Clark, 1997; Watson & Tellegen, 1985) have typically characterized positive affectivity as "one's level of pleasurable engagement with the environment."

Multiple studies have shown that positive emotions/affects have a wide range of effects on individuals (Lyubomirsky, King, & Diener, 2005; Pressman & Cohen, 2005). Positive affectivity has found to be a good predictor of health and better prognosis form illness. It has been generally found that people with high level of positive affectivity had longer life span, fewer pains and symptoms of illness, for example ,blood pressure ,and are less vulnerable to viral diseases, such as common cold (Cohen & Pressman, 2006). Individuals high in PA view the world in a more positive light and report leading full and interesting lives (Watson & Pennebaker, 1989). It has also been shown that individuals who are better at coping with stress may handle stressful situations by activating or maintaining positive emotions (Tugade, Fredrickson, & Barrett, 2004). Research shows that PA relate to different classes of variables, such as social activity and the frequency of pleasant events. PA provides a psychological break or respite from stress, supporting continuing efforts to replenish resources depleted by stress (Lazarus, 1991; Khosla, 2006). High PA reflects enthusiasm, high energy, concentration, determination and pleasurable engagement (McIntyre, Watson, Clark, & Cross, 1991), whereas low PA is characterized by sadness and lethargy. Its buffering functions provide a useful antidote to the problem associated with negative emotions and ill health due to stress (Fredrickson, 2001). Positive affect promoted coping responses which led to finding meaning in various stressful experiences (Khosla, 2006).

OPTIMISM

Optimism as having "hopefulness and confidence about the future or successful outcome of something; a tendency to take a favorable or hopeful view." The word is originally derived from the Latin optimum, meaning "best." Optimism is the propensity to look at the bright side of any situation and expect the best possible outcome from any series of events. People who feel optimism live their lives expecting positive outcomes and events. Optimism is an individual difference variable that reflects the extent to which people hold generalized favorable expectancies for their future. Higher levels of optimism have been related prospectively to better subjective well-being in times of adversity or difficulty (Carver, Scheier, & Segerstrom, 2010). Optimism is defined as positive outcome expectancies, either of a generalized, dispositional nature or with regard to a specific situation.

Optimism is the most focused positive psychological construct in current researches relating psychological state to health and illness (Seligman & Csikszentmihalyi, 2000). This construct has been defined in two different ways. The first approach emphasizes the optimistic explanatory style (Abramson, Seligman, & Teasdale, 1978; Peterson & Seligman, 1988). This view of optimism is in contrast to learned helplessness and sense of uncontrollability. The second approach conceptualizes the optimism as personality disposition (Scheier & Carver, 1985). Cohen et al. (1999), for example, demonstrated that whether dispositional optimism was associated with better or worse immune responding depended on whether participants faced chronic or acute stressors. Whereas optimism was associated with better immune responding among people facing more acute stressors, it was associated with worse immune responding among people facing more chronic stressors. Dispositional optimism refers to generalized outcome expectation that good things, rather than bad things, will happen. Dispositional optimism and situational optimism has been found to be positively associated with good mental as well as physical health status (DeMoor et al., 2006). According to Scheier & Carver (1985), it a trait of an equilibrated personality, in time and in various situations, that influences the way in which individuals come to terms with present, past and future events in life. Dispositional optimism has been reported to be negatively associated with depression and anxiety (Schou et al., 2004), distress (Epping-Jorden et al., 1999) and positively associated with better psychological adjustment in spite of higher successful life events (Cozzarelli, (1993). This view upholds optimism as personality trait of generalize expectancies concerning future outcomes.

Optimistic individuals are positive about events in daily life. In the research carried out regarding this perspective, positive correlations have been found between optimism and physical/mental well-being. They think that they can avoid problems in daily life and prevent them from happening, and therefore they cope with stressful situations more successfully than pessimists (Aspinwall, Richter & Hoffman, 2001; Peterson & Avila, 1995). Optimistic subjects tend to have more frequently protective attitudes are more resilient to stress and are inclined to use more appropriate coping strategies. Optimists believe that positive events are more stable and frequent than negative ones.

The present chapter was aimed to explaining the brief introduction of the study and description of the concepts used in the present study. In the next chapter statement of the problem; Rational of the present study, objectives and hypotheses will be discussed.

Chapter-II

REVIEW OF LITERATURE

This review summarizes the empirical literature concerned with the relationship between stress, personal or psychological attributes and health status. Various personal variables are operationalized and reviewed systematically.

In last few decades numerous studies have been conducted to examine the relationship between stress and health and its effects on employee's behavior. But there were no such studies available where resilience, optimism and positive affectivity has been taken as moderator variables of stress and health relationship. Perhaps, with a wide range of research coverage on resilience literature relating it to children and adolescents, only few studies have been investigated resilience among adults and old people. Therefore more researches are required to draw a conclusive fact about resilience, optimism and positive affectivity among them.

Studies related to Stress and Health

Throughout the life, our physical and mental health are impacted by a host of biological, psychological, and social variables. For example, it is now fairly clear that several distal variables including the physical environment (e.g., built environment, noise, crowding), community/ neighboring (Wanders man & Nation, 1998), culture (Hruschka, 2009), as well as various other more major (e.g., cataclysmic events, major life events, ambient stressors; Monroe, 2008; Wanders man & Nation, 1998) and minor stressors (Kohn, Lafreniere, & Gurevich, 1990) have the potential, depending in part on how we appraise any event or environment, to affect us negatively (Lazarus & Folkman, 1984). Early studies have revealed that daily hassles related stress such as conflicts with family members or colleagues, work problems, time pressure, or financial difficulties were inversely related to psychological and physical health (Banez & Compas, 1990; Selongis, Folkman, & Lazarus, 1988; Lai, 1995; Lai, Hamid, & Chow, 1996; Majella de Jong et al., 1996). According to Almeida (2005), daily hassles related stress not only affect well-being by having immediate and direct impact on emotional and physical functioning, but also by piling up over a number of days to create persistent irritations and frustrations.

Researchers have investigated the stress–illness connection by quantifying life stress in terms of life changes or life events. Life changes are sources of stress because they force us to adjust. They include both positive events, such as getting married and negative events, such as the death of a loved one. Evidence shows that people who experience greater numbers of life changes are more likely to suffer from psychological and physical health problems (Dohrenwend, 2006). At the same time, demographic markers such as age and sex (Yount, Hoddinott, & Stein, 2010), social support (Cohen, 2004), coping (Lazarus & Folkman, 1984), as well as various risk-related and preventive health behaviors may also contribute by attenuating or exacerbating the impact of stress on health (Hagger-Johnson, Mõttus, Craig, & Starr, 2012). Acute episodic stressful life events have been identified as a risk factor for disease including breast cancer (Lillberg, Verkasalo, Kaprio, Teppo, Helenius, & Koskenvuo, 2003). Any sources of stress not only diminish our capacity for adjustment, but also may adversely affect our health. It has been noticed that people are unhappy in their lives fall sick more in comparison to those who are happy and enjoy life.

The relationship between stress and health may be traced back in the Cannon's (1914) work on homeostasis. He described stress as a disturbed emotional state which puts detrimental impact on physiological functioning. In 1960s Holmes and Rahe reported that naturally accruing or induced stress evokes significant alterations in the functioning of most bodily tissues, organs, and systems. These changes in turn lead to a lowering of the body's resistance to disease by suppressing immune system. Stress has been associated with poor health in individuals across the lifespan and in many cultures (Lin & Ensel, 1989; Marmot & Wilkinson, 1999). Stress is a risk factor for a wide variety of disease (Cohen, Janicki-Deverts, & Miller, 2007; McEwen, 1998). Stress has also been linked to health indicators such as obesity (measured through indices such as body mass index and percentage body fat), high systolic blood pressure, and elevated heart rates (Bell, Summerson, Spangler, & Konen, 2001; Brand, Hanson, & Godaert, 2000). A growing body of research suggests that stress is detrimental to mental and physical well-being (Majella de Jong, timmerman, & Emmelkamp, 1996; Fabricarore et al., 2004).

There is also convincing evidence to show that stress can produce changes in the immune system and increase the chances of someone becoming ill. According to Kemeny & Schedlowski, (2007) occasional stress may not impair our health, chronic or repetitive stress can eventually weaken the body's immune system. A weakened immune system increases our susceptibility to many illnesses, including the common cold and the flu, and may increase the risk of developing chronic diseases, including cancer. Stress has been implicated in the development of cardiovascular disorders, high blood pressures, as well as psychosomatic disorders including ulcers, asthma allergies and headaches. Chronic stress can damage our health, leaving us more vulnerable to a range of diseases and other physical health problems. Chronic stress also has been identified as a risk factor for a variety of diseases including cardiovascular disease, asthma, infectious disease, stroke, cancer, ulcers and rheumatoid arthritis (Anderson, Kiecolt-Glaser, & Glaser, 1994, Chandola, et.al, 2008; Cohen & Williamson, 1991, Karasek, Baker, Marxer, Ahlbom, & Theorell, 1981; Sandberg, et al., 2000). For example, in a prospective study that included participants from the Whitehall Study, Chandola and colleagues, (2008) reported that individuals who experienced chronic work stress, had a 68% greater risk of heart disease at the 14 year follow up than individuals who were not in enduring stress.

Researchers estimated that stress plays an important role in 50-70% of all physical illnesses. Studies also reveal that 60% of medical visits are primarily for stress related symptoms. It was found that many visits to physicians, perhaps even most, can be traced to stress-related illness. Stress is associated with an increased risk of various types of physical illness, ranging from digestive disorders to heart disease. The field of psychoneuroimmunology studies relationships between psychological factors, especially stress, and the workings of the endocrine system, the immune system, and the nervous system (Kiecolt-Glaser et al., 2002). When stress is prolonged, it affects physical health and impairs psychological functioning. Health professionals have long recognized the negative effects of stress upon psychological and physical health. Psychological stressors can dampen the response of the immune system, especially when the stress is intense or prolonged (Segerstrom & Miller, 2004). Scientists recently discovered that one way chronic stress damages the body's immune system is by increasing levels of a chemical in the body called interleukin-6 (Kiecolt Glaser et al., 2003). Sustained high levels of this chemical are linked to inflammation, which in turn can contribute to the development of many disorders, including cardiovascular disease, cancer, and arthritis.

Stress-health relationship is so robust and universal that it has been observed in infants, children, adolescents, young adults, adults and the elderly (Graham, Christian, & Kiecolt-Glaser, 2006). It has been reported consistently that people with easy-going disposition show stress-resistance. Studies have shown that excessive stress during the teen years can have a negative impact upon both physical and mental health later in life. For example, teen stress is a risk factor for the development of depression, a serious condition that carries an increases risk of suicide. Individuals may be more susceptible to the negative effects of stress on health if they are from difficult childhood environment responses to stressors (Hanson & Chen, 2010). The instabilities of human system create psychological and/or biological changes, which places individuals at an increased risk for poor health (Cohen et al., 1997).

Studies related to Occupational Stress and Health

Occupational stress is a universal phenomenon that is associated with several deleterious consequences such as negative physical and mental health outcomes (Kakiashvili, Leszek, and Rutkowski, 2013) and a number of negative organizational outcomes such as impaired work performance and high turnover (Bridger, Day, and Morton, 2013). Occupational stress might be harmful for physiological and psychological effects on workers. Occupational stress occurs primarily in response to how an individual appraises an occupational stressor (Ashkanasy, Ashton-James, and Jordan, 2004) and there are individual differences in how people engage in this process of appraisal (FinlayJones, 2014). High work-related stress can lead to impaired work performance, and chronic stress may impair attention (Skosnik, Chatterton, Swisher, and Park, 2000) and decision-making skills (Starcke and Brand, 2012). Furthermore, it has been reported that job related stress is "a major contribution of the six leading causes of death in the United States: coronary heart disease, cancer, lung ailments, accidental injuries, cirrhosis of the liver and suicide" (Tipgos, 1987). Individuals exposed to continued or high levels of stress, develop strain reactions which may be psychological, physical, behavioral or organizational (Ivancevich & Mattesom, 1984; Mroczek & Almeida, 2004). Some researchers in organizational stress have mainly focused on emotional, behavioral and health outcomes of stress experienced by the workers (Brief, Schuler, & Van Sell, 1981; Cooper & Marshall, 1976: Ivansevich & Matteson, 1980; Cotton & Hart, 2003). Marcia Maurer (2002) stated that stress-induced illnesses are prevalent in the workplace today, and stress is the problem of the sufferer and the employer. However, for some workers and under some circumstances, they might translate into poor performance at work into other psychological and social problem and into poor physical health (Devereux, Buckle, & Vlchonikolis, 1999).

The structure of the organization itself can also be a source of stress for employees. For example, hierarchical, top-down management structures that provide workers with little or no say in the decision-making process, restrictions on behavior, office politics, lack of effective consultation (Cooper & Marshall, 1976), and erratic working hours (Greenhaus & Parasuraman, 1987) can all have detrimental effects on workers' well-being. Workplace stress can have a wide-ranging and negative impact on the health and well-being of the individual and his or her day to day functioning. This is observable at physical level (e.g., exhaustion, headaches, high blood pressure), at psychological level (e.g., depression, anxiety, low self-esteem) and at cognitive level.

Devidson, Cooper and Baldini (1995) examined levels of occupational stress among graduate managers (126 female and 220 male) in UK. Comparison of male and female managers on occupational stress variables revealed that female graduate managers scored significantly higher pressure scores on all seven sources of pressure subscales, including the added gender factor related to discrimination and prejudice. While females were more likely than males to adopt positive coping strategies, they were more at risk of mental and physical ill-health along with lower overall job satisfaction scores; particularly those in junior and middle management positions. Multivariate analyses disclosed that predictors of physical ill-health, mental health and job dissatisfaction were often quite dissimilar for male and females.

Mishra et al., (1997) conducted a study to compare the occupational stress among public and private sector public relations officers. The occupational stress index (A.K. Srivastava and A.P. Singh, 1981) was administered to the sample population. Critical ratio test was used to find out the difference between perceived occupational stress among public and private sector public relations officers. The analysis of the data revealed that public relations officers of public sector experienced significantly higher occupational stress on the dimensions of role ambiguity, role conflict, unreasonable group and political pressures, powerlessness, poor peer relations at work, intrinsic impoverishment, low status and strenuous working condition as compared to public relations officers of private sector. Second, no significant difference was found between the PRO's of public and private sector on the dimensions of responsibility for persons, under participation and unprofitability.

A number of studies have found that occupational stressors such as heavy job demands and lack of control are associated with various health problems for women. High-strain jobs have been linked with psychological distress, pain, and reduced physical functioning among nurses (Amick et al., 1998, Bourbonnais, comeau, & Vezina, 1999).

Evans and Steptoe (2002) investigated the association of work stress, types of work and gender-role orientation with psychological well-being and sickness absence on a sample consisted of men and women occupying jobs where they were in cultural and numerical minority. Female accountants were more likely than other group to have high anxiety and depression scores, while male nurses had the highest rates of sickness absence. Male nurses and female accountants also reported more work-related hassles than did female nurses and male accountants. The results suggest that when men and women occupy jobs in which they are in cultural and numerical minority, there may be adverse health effects that are gender-specific. Psychological traits related to socially constructed gender roles may also be relevant, and mediate in part the differences in psychological well-being between men and women.

Aziz (2003) investigated the prevalence of organizational role stress among Indian information technology employees. The study reported more stress among men as compared to women. Aditya and Sen (1993) compared the level of stress between men and women executives in India. Results shows that male and female executives differed significantly on role ambiguity, role conflict, inter-role distance, future prospects, and human relations at work, femininity and masculinity dimensions. Authors discussed the results in terms of greater reluctance to self-disclose among men, different socialization patterns for men and women.

Harris, Cumming and Campbell (2006) studied workplace stress, general perceived stress, psychological distress and life satisfaction among 139 health professionals. Compared with expectations based on normative data, more people in the present sample had depression, anxiety and stress scores in the mild, moderate, severe, or very severe range. The single significant predictor of psychological distress and life satisfaction was perceived stress.

Sackeya and Sanda (2009) examined the existing relationships among job characteristics, symptoms of stress, and the development of health outcomes (depression, anxiety and physical symptoms) among women in lower and middle management positions (n=170) in organizations in Ghana. Data were analyzed from interviews and questionnaires, viz. occupational stress indicator, the depression, anxiety and stress scale, and the Beck's anxiety inventory. Results indicated that managerial women experience a number of work-related stressors which produce strain symptoms that function as predictors of their ill-health in organizations. It was concluded that since work-related stressors are predictors of women managers' ill-health in the work environment, organizations should be aware of the stressors in order to be able to guard against the deterioration of job performances of their women managers.

Sandmark, (2011) studied 16 females chosen from a cohort of 300 females that held full-time white-collar jobs in high level positions usually dominated by men. Their study was interested in the long-term sick leave in female white-collar workers that resulted from burnout and stress-related illnesses. Results showed that females with work stress experienced inequality, higher expectations than their male counterparts, mismatch between competence and job demands. The imbalance in work and private life contributed to the exposure of long term external and internal stress that manifested as overexertion.

Kang and Sandhu, (2012) taken a sample of 316 bank branch managers from public and private sector banks operating in the state of Punjab (India) to examined the relationship between job and family related stressors and the physical and mental health of bank branch managers. In the results a significant number of the respondents have been found experiencing poor physical and mental health. Sources of stress like, 'Highly intricate nature of the job', 'lack of time for family and personal care', 'insufficient training and career uncertainties', 'performance constraints and pressures', 'surveillance required', 'unwanted criticism', 'travelling and transfers', and 'family obligations', have been found affecting the physical and mental health of bank branch managers.

Fan, Blumenthal, Watkins, & Sherwood, (2015) examine the impact of psychosocial stress at work and at home on anxiety and depression among medically healthy employed men and women (n= 129, aged 30–60). Data were analyzed by Beck Depression Inventory-II (BDI-II), and anxiety symptoms, measured using the Spielberger Trait Anxiety Inventory (STAI). Psychosocial stress at work was measured using the Job Content Questionnaire to assess job psychological demands, job control, job social support and job insecurity. Psychosocial stress at home was assessed by 12 questions including stress at home, personal problems, family demands and feelings about home life. Results revealed that work and home stress were significantly and strongly associated with anxiety and depression symptoms in both men and women.

In addition, however, we have included the dispositional variables like resilience, optimism and positive affectivity as important additional explanatory constructs in stress and health research.

Resilience and Health

With the early investigation of the concept during 1950s made a shift in the paradigm of research from 'risk-research' to 'resilience research' by the beginning of 1980s (Boyden & Cooper, 2007). Now a day, the concept of resilience is being employed with a wide range of scientific disciplines ranging from developmental psychology, ecological economics, social policy genetics and disaster studies (Boyend & Coper, 2007; Bartley, 2006; Brand & Jax, 2007). Today the theme of resilience in the literature is wide spread and only a short and limited overview of the resilience research at time is hardly possible. Very few previous researches have been conducted with pre-adolescent and younger children (Garmezy, Masten, & Tellegen, 1984; Masten et al., 1988;

Werner & Smith, 1982) or with young adults (Rutter & Quinton, 1984; Werner, 1989). Most studies often associate the concept of resilience with extreme or adverse stress, traumatic events or loss (DiCorcia & Tronick, 2011; Schetter & Dolbier, 2011) with more focus on children and adolescents and less on adults (Jackson, Firtko, & Edenborough, 2007; Kitano & Lewis, 2005; Wagnild & Young, 1993). Perhaps, with a wide range of research coverage on resilience relating it to several illness and health related psycho-social factors, there are several gaps identified in the existing literature and there is a lack of comparative studies. All these perspectives present important exciting areas for further research to better understand how people cope with adversities.

The most prominent feature of 'risk-resilience' transition is the researches in the area of health covering a wide range of topics: chronic illness (Bellin & Kovacs, 2006), child mortality (Garenne & Gakusi, 2006), mental and physical disabilities (Retzlaff et al., 2006), stress (Joiner et al., 2005) and poor health in old age (Walter-Ginzberg et al., 2005; Gattuso, 2003). However, most importantly, risk factor do not predict a negative consequence, they simply expose the individual to a condition involving a higher incidence of negative outcomes. Resilience involves individual variations in response to risk in the way that poor outcomes are reduced or good outcomes are enhanced (Rutter, 1987). The mechanism involved in the resilience in presence of risk factors remains a topic which is not properly explored and is an issue for debate. However, undoubtedly, there exist complex interactions of individual and environmental factors that promote resilience (Rutter, 1993).

Psychological resilience is a relatively stable personality characteristic that is thought to be characterized by the ability to bounce back and adapt to negative experiences (Block & Block, 1980; Block & Kremen, 1996). Psychological resilience has been defined as the ability of a person to recover, re-bound, bounce-back, adjust or even thrive following misfortune, change or adversity (Garcia-Dia et al., 2013) and is widely acknowledged to be a complex, dynamic and multi-dimensional phenomenon (Waugh and Koster, 2014). An important issue in the health-resilience literature is its protective nature, which helps individuals to cope with adversity. Resilience plays the important role of a protective factor, protecting the individual's psychological being and increasing positive changes when coping with stressful situations (Dolbier, Jaggars, & Steinhardt, 2010; Kinman & Grant, 2011). It seeks to promote and maintain health and prevent illness (Muller, 2009).

Studies have now shown a link between psychological resilience and various health outcomes such as burnout, secondary traumatic stress, depression, and anxiety (Mak et al., 2011; Mealer et al., 2012; McGarry et al., 2013). For example, a study by Mealer et al. (2012) included 744 intensive care nurses working in the United States and found that high resilience was associated with a lower prevalence of burnout, symptoms of anxiety and depression and symptoms of post-traumatic stress disorder. Similarly, a study by McGarry et al. (2013) conducted in Australia with health professionals working in a pediatric hospital, found that high resilience was associated with lower prevalence of burnout, symptoms of anxiety and depression and symptoms of post-traumatic stress disorder and low psychological resilience was associated with higher secondary traumatic stress.

Resilience is a construct that can be applied to children, adolescents, adults, and the elderly across different ethnic and socio-economic backgrounds (Belgrave et al., 2000; Connell, Spencer, & Aber, 1994; Ripple & Luthar, 2000; Smith & Carlson, 1997; Smokowski, Reynolds, & Bezruczko, 2000; Waller et al., 2003). Coping with painful events and unpleasant emotions is a struggle for every human-being. Those who are less resilient may turn to unhealthy actions or negative beliefs about themselves to cope with the difficulties encountered in their lives (Smokowski, 1999). Resilience can be defined as positively coping with stressful events (Smokowski et al., 1999), or adaptive coping in the face of multiple risk factors (Waller et al., 2003). The various components of resilience can also be thought of having a "buffering" effect between risk factors and negative life outcomes. Research on resilience focuses on those individuals who have overcome difficult life circumstances and have become successful, as well as what factors promote such adaptive functioning.

Ong and colleagues (2006) found that self-reported trait resilience contributed to both stress resistance and recovery processes. Successful adaptation in the face of stress is a process that is beneficial for all individuals; however, not everyone can produce positive affect during stressful times. Therefore, an important task for researchers is to determine whether there are certain psychological factors that might serve to promote positive affect and these resilience processes. Research has consistently shown that resilient individuals have optimistic outlooks on life, are open to new experiences, and have higher positive emotionality (Block & Kremen, 1996). Resilient individuals use positive emotions more frequently and may be able to access these emotions during times of stress (Tugade & Fredrickson, 2007). It is possible, then, that highly resilient individuals may be more likely to use positive emotions in resilience processes. One important characteristic of trait resilience is having an optimistic outlook on life (Block & Kremen, 1996). As a component of trait resilience, it is possible that dispositional optimism may also influence resilience processes in a similar manner. For example, individuals high in trait optimism may be more likely to generate positive affect during stressful experiences that, in turn, can be utilized to bolster resistance to, and recovery from stress. Resilience is a relatively stable personality trait characterized by the ability to overcome, steer through, and bounce back from adversity (Block & Kremen, 1996; Block & Block, 1980).

Recent research, moreover, suggests that positive emotions are a crucial component of trait resilience (Tugade & Fredrickson, 2004; Tugade, Fredrickson, & Barrett, 2004). Rather than being a simple by product of resilience, however, the experience of positive emotion is thought to have adaptive benefits in the coping process (for reviews, see Folkman & Moskowitz, 2000a, & 2004). Empirical support for this prediction comes from research demonstrating that resilient individuals tend to draw on positive emotion-eliciting coping strategies such as benefit finding and positive reappraisal (Affleck & Tennen, 1996; Folkman & Moskowitz, 2000b), humor and infusing ordinary events with positive meaning (Folkman, Moskowitz, Ozer, & Park, 1997; Ong et al., 2006), and goal-directed problem-focused coping (Billings, Folkman, Acree, & Moskowitz, 2000; Folkman, 1997) to regulate negative emotional experiences. Taken as a whole, these findings indicate that traits (e.g., psychological resilience) with functional properties associated with positive emotions may serve to strengthen resistance to stress by affording greater access to positive emotional resources (Ong & Bergeman, 2004a; Tugade et al., 2004), which, in turn, may help to provide a momentary respite from ongoing stressful experiences (Folkman & Moskowitz, 2000a; Zautra, Johnson, & Davis, 2005).

According to Ekas and Whitman, (2011) individuals high in trait resilience, positive affect served as a protective factor to help resist the negative effects of stress, and this effect was found on both high and low stress days. It is defined as "the process of, capacity for or outcome of successful adaptation despite challenging or threatening circumstances" (Masten et al., 1990, p. 426). This definition implies that two critical conditions must be met: (1) there must be exposure to significant adversity; and (2) there must be successful adaptation despite threats to well-being. In other words, resilience cannot occur without exposure to some level of risk; however, the level of risk that is necessary to deem an individual's positive adaptation as resilient is unclear (Cummings, Davies, & Campbell, 2002; Luthar, Cichetti, & Becker, 2000). Early resilience research initially characterized those identified as resilient as being remarkable, rare, extraordinary, or special (e.g. Masten, 2001). Recent research, however, has shown that resilience in the face of loss (e.g. death of loved one) or severe trauma (e.g. September 11, 2001 terrorist attacks) is more common than previously thought (Bonanno, 2004). Furthermore, successful adaptation can be achieved through a variety of different resilience processes.

In a series of coordinated experimental and individual difference studies, Fredrickson and colleagues (Fredrickson et al., 2003; Tugade et al., 2004) found that high-resilient individuals exhibited faster physiological and emotional recovery from stress. In one study (Tugade et al., 2004) higher trait resilience was linked to quicker cardiovascular recovery following a laboratory stressor. In another study (Fredrickson et al., 2003), higher trait resilience was associated with lower subsequent depressive symptoms. Older individuals are at higher risk for many diseases, both acute and chronic (Hawkley & Cacioppo, 2010; Smith et al., 2003). In addition, older adults may be especially likely to experience certain psychosocial stressors, such as spousal caregiving and bereavement (Moss, Moss, & Hansson, 2001). Maddi (1999) found that hardy, resilient employees in a firm undergoing a massive downsizing maintained their health, happiness, and performance; Larson and Luthans (2006) found the factory workers' resiliency related to their job satisfaction; and Youssef and Luthans, (2007) found that employees' level of resilience related to their satisfaction, commitment, and happiness.

Because of negative life events and chronic life conditions are more likely to accumulate with age, studies are needed that clarify how certain older adults are able to maintain and regain emotional health in the face of ongoing stress (Ong & Bergeman, 2004). A related gap in the literature is the relative dearth of daily process studies that track the real-world adaptation processes of individuals, particularly older adults, intensively over time (Almeida, 2005; Mroczek, Spiro, & Almeida, 2003). Additionally needed, therefore, are studies that sharpen understanding of the ways in which older adults effectively negotiate stressors in their everyday lives (Mroczek & Spiro, 2007). Finally, extant studies of resilience, from childhood to old age, have given limited attention to the dynamic interplay between process and trait conceptualizations of resilience (Block & Kremen, 1996; Luthar, Cicchetti, & Becker, 2000). Crucially needed are empirical investigations that further elucidate how stable personality traits influence and support meaningful short-term adaptation to stress (Fleeson, 2004) and improve health. Several studies on nurses (Mealer et al., 2012) and doctors (Taku, 2014) found resilience was a protective factor that can buffer the relationship between risk factors and burnout. Furthermore, the mediating effect of resilience on life events/learning stress and learning burnout of students (Wang and Zhang, 2011; Zhang, 2013) and the moderating effect of resilience on role stress and job burnout of teachers (Xu, Zhang, Sun, & Tian, 2013) have been proved.

In a recent study on role of trauma exposure and anxiety disorders in adult women, Scali et al. (2012) found that women scoring high in the 10-Items Connor-Davidson Resilience Scale (CD-RISC-10) were less likely than women scoring low in the CD-RISC-10 to develop anxiety and mood disorders. They linked resilience and lifetime trauma exposure and found that the variables are influenced by the self-evaluation of resilience by the women faced with current stressful situations and the different perception of stress. They further commented that individuals with some history of lifetime low or moderate adversity are better adjusted with healthy well-being in recent adverse events than individuals with no history of adversity and high adversity. The concept concurs with the idea that resilience grows with successful process of coping in adversity and leads to a better psychological functioning and well-being (Scali et al., 2012; van Heugten, 2013). In the same way, resilience in work stress is able to buffer against negative effects of stress and improve the working employees' well-being.

In a recent study of relationships among positive emotions, coping, resilience and mental health on a sample of 200 postdoctoral research fellows was found that the broaden-and-build theory in that positive emotions may enhance resilience directly as well as indirectly through the mediating role of coping strategies—particularly via adaptive coping. Resilience also moderated the association of stress with trait anxiety and depressive symptoms (Gloria & Steinhardt, 2014).

In a study the mediating and moderating effect in the relationship between resilience, stress and burnout among 541 civil servants of Beijing, China was found that resilience was a moderator between work stress and burnout, and it could serve as a buffer to mitigate the adverse effects of work stress. These results suggest that resilience could be a positive personality trait for alleviating or eliminating work stress and combating burnout of civil servants of Beijing (Hao, Hong, Xu, Zhou & Xie, 2015).

Optimism and Health

Positive variables can play an important role in coping with the condition and in determining the outcome of disease. Optimism is an important personality variable with respect to behavioral health outcomes. Scheier and Carver, 1987 define optimism as ''general expectations that good things will happen'' (p. 172). It is a relatively stable, generalized expectation that positive outcomes will occur across important life domains. Optimism also benefits people's actions and their potential to achieve in times of adversity, according to Scheier and Carver, 1992. There is evidence that optimistic people present a higher quality of life compared to those with low levels of optimism or even pessimists. Optimism may significantly influence mental and physical well-being by the promotion of a healthy lifestyle as well as by adaptive behaviors and cognitive responses, associated with greater flexibility, problem-solving capacity and a more efficient elaboration of negative information (Conversano et al., 2010).

Optimism in the literature has been defined in several ways– as a disposition, a situation construct, an attribution style, a cognitive bias, or a pervasive illusion (Gilbert, Fiske, & Lindzey, 1998). Optimism can be explained as a quite stable component of the explanatory style adopted by a person in interpreting life events through causal attributions (Abramson, Seligman, & Teasdale, 1978; Peterson, Schulman, Castellon, & Seligman, 1992). Taylor and Gollwitzer (1995) assert that optimism serves as an important resource in the goal attainment process and act as important resource in supporting efforts towards goal achievement. Considerable volume of research demonstrated that optimism is associated with better mental health and better psychological adjustment in clinical sample (Ringdal et al., 1996; Schulz et al., 1996) as well as non-clinical samples (Robinson-Whelen et al., 1997; Segerstrom et al., 1998). For example, pre surgery optimism predicts higher quality of life and life satisfaction 8 months after coronary artery bypass surgery (Fitzgerald, Tennen, Affleck, & Pransky, 1993). A more recent meta-analysis (Nes & Segerstrom, 2006 p, 235) found that optimism leads to the use of more approach coping ("strategies aiming to eliminate, reduce, or manage stressors or emotions") and less avoidance coping ("seeking to ignore, avoid, or withdraw from stressor).

High level optimism, on the contrast, relates with better physiological and functional measures of physical health. In several prospective studies, optimism was found as a baseline predictor of later well-being. Optimism not only helps individuals adapt to stressful events more successfully, it also protect health (Taylor, Kemeny, Bower, Gruenewald, & Reed, 2000). Higher levels of optimism have been related prospectively to better subjective well-being in times of adversity or difficulty (Carver, Scheier, & Segerstrom, 2010). Mostly studies on optimism emphasized on the cognitive aspects. However, in human information processing system, emotions, motivations, and cognitive processes also coexist. Eventually, subjective experience is ultimately shaped by the complex interplay of these factors in short and long term.

Scheier et al., (1989) conducted a study on men underwent coronary artery bypass graft (CABG) to investigate the relationship between optimism and change in enzyme and EKG as indicative of myocardial infraction during surgery. They reported that the higher level of optimism was correlated with the fewer enzyme and EKG changes. Along with this they also concluded that patients with higher degree of optimism recovered quicker and experienced less functional disability for at least six months after surgery.

Research has shown that optimism can correlate with good health at many stages, including preventative health (making it less likely to experience illness). Severity a duration of illness, and reduction of relapse chances. However, Affleck, Tennen, and Apter (2001) Studied optimism and health in terms of physical symptoms, coping strategies and negative affect for those suffering from rheumatoid arthritis, asthma, and fibromyalgia.

Subjective aspects of the quality of life and psychological health, optimism and happiness at greater extent may contribute to the onset and maintenance of anxiety, depression and other psychoses, which designate risk factor for the psychosomatic disorders (Frasure-Smith & Lesperance, 2005).

In two years follow-up study of aging men optimism was found to predict higher levels of general health perception, validity, mental health and lower level of bodily pain (Achat, Kawachi, Spiro, DeMolles, & Sparrow, 2000). A large body of research on patient with suffering from chronic disease has provided the evidence that optimism is linked to better survival and adaptation (Allison, Guichard, fung, & Gilain, 2003; Symister & Friend, 2003).

A large volume of related literature documented the role of optimism in better survival and adaptation among patients with chronic disease (Allison, Guichard, Fung, & Gilian, 2003; Fitzerald, Tennen, Affleck, & Pransky, 1993; Fournier, DeRidder, & Bensing, 2002; Maruta, Colligan, Malinchoc, & Offord, 2000; Scheier, et al., 1999; Symister & Friend, 2003). Moreover, to draw any strong conclusion on the basis of existing literature on optimism and health will be too early for putting step forward meant for an immature conclusion.

There are few studies reporting non-significant and even inverse relationship between optimism and health. For example, Chesterman, Cohen, & Adler (1990) found that optimism was associated with more birth complications in women got pregnant at later age.

Studies demonstrated that optimism is substantially correlated with self-mastery, neuroticism, anxiety, and self-esteem, whereas, the predictive ability of optimism for depression and certain coping strategies remain to be well established after controlling the overlapping with these variables (Scheier, Carver, & Bridges, 1994). Along with this functional versus harmful effects of optimistic beliefs have been raised persistently (Block & Colvin, 1994; Taylor & Brown, 1994).

Mostly studies do not attempt to manipulate happiness and optimism showing direct and lasting effect on physical health. Fairly good volume of findings represent the fact that cheerfulness as an indicative of good moods are related with healthier life style, at least over the short period of time (Salovey, Rothman, & Steward. 2000). However, such type of findings does not mean that good mood always lead to good health. There is growing evidence that optimism is associated with greater physical and mental health (Achat, Kawachi, Spiro, DeMolles, & Sparrow, 2000; Scheier & Carver, 1992; Segerstrom, Taylor, Kemeny, & Fahey, 1998).

Optimism and perceived control are two such characteristics that have been associated with increased well-being (e.g. Scheier & Carver, 1992). Indeed, Optimistic patients exhibit faster recovery from cardiac bypass surgery (Scheier et al., 1989), and are more likely to employ positive health practices (Scheier & Carver, 1992).

Another study Segerstrom et al., (1998) determined that situational optimism was a stronger predictor of mood than dispositional optimism and predicted immune changes when dispositional optimism did not. Segerstrom et al., (1998) explain that there exists a growing body of evidence that elucidates the relationship of optimism and other psychosocial factors to biological processes associated with physical health. It is recognized that optimistic attitude that is, the expectation that good things will happen, seems to promote a higher level of physical and psychological well-being (Scheier, Carver & Bridges, 1994). Optimism as inherent aspects of human nature converge with empirical investigations of it as an individual difference to show that optimism can be a highly beneficial psychological characteristic linked to good mood, achievement, and physical health.

Many studies have found that optimism is correlated with better physical well-being compared to pessimism. Moreover, in contrast with optimism, pessimism is correlated with excessive somatic complaints. In a study on a population of elderly subjects of both sexes, aged between 65-85 years, Giltay et al., (2004) noted that dispositional optimism predicted less probability of mortality in general and of cardiovascular mortality in particular. These data have been confirmed in a subsequent longitudinal study on a population of males aged between 64 - 84 years in which an inverse correlation was reported between dispositional optimism and the risk of cardiovascular death Giltay et al., (2006).

Matthews et al., (2010) observed that in the three years following the menopause, carotid atherosclerosis tended to progress more slowly in optimistic women compared to their pessimistic peers.

In reference to oncological patients, Schulz et al., (1996) noted that high scores on the pessimism items of the LOT (a measure of dispositional optimism) significantly predicted premature death in young patients with breast cancer. Optimistic individuals are positive about events in daily life. In the research carried out regarding this perspective, positive correlations have been found between optimism and physical/mental well-being. Optimistic subjects tend to have more frequently protective attitudes are more resilient to stress and are inclined to use more appropriate coping strategies (Scheier & Carver, 1985). Among patients with neck or head cancer, optimists manifested significantly greater survival a year after diagnosis when compared to pessimists (Scheier & Carver, 1987).

People with optimistic explanatory style tend to enjoy good health. Optimism helps in sustaining immune functions under stress (Segerstrom et. al, 1998). Scheier and Carver (1985) and Scheier, Carver and Bridges (2001) noted that people expecting best and looking bright side of the things reported less fatigue, fewer aches, pains and minor illness. They also noted that optimists tend to have better mental and physical health and recover more quickly when they become ill.

Positive and negative expectations regarding the future are important for understanding the vulnerability to mental disorders, in particular mood and anxiety disorders, as well as to physical illness. A significant positive relation emerges between optimism and coping strategies focused on social support and emphasis on positive aspects of stressful situations. Through employment of specific coping strategies, optimism exerts an indirect influence also on the quality of life. There is evidence that optimistic people present a higher quality of life compared to those with low levels of optimism or even pessimists. (Conversano, Rotondo, Lensi, Vista, Arpone, & Reda, 2010).

In relation to this, Van der Velden et al., (2007) have studied the association between 'dispositional optimism' and depression in victims of a natural disaster. The results of this research show that compared to optimists, pessimists nurtured little hope for the future and were more at risk for depressive and anxiety disorders, with subsequent impairment of social functioning and quality of life. The role of optimism in the quality of life has also been investigated in depressive disorders emerging in patients suffering from somatic pathologies, (such as acute coronary syndrome, for instance) in which a significant inverse correlation was found between dispositional optimism and level of satisfaction in life on one hand and depressive symptoms emerging after the cardiovascular event on the other hand (Steele & Wade, 2004).

Giltay et al., (2006) raised the question of using psychotherapy to promote an optimistic disposition in pessimistic subjects, thus developing an efficient strategy to fight depression. Evidence regarding this subject has emerged also from studies carried out on victims of catastrophic events such as natural disasters. In fact, it has been observed that even one single session of cognitive-behavioral therapy, targeted at enhancing the sense of control and coping with incapacitating disturbances that ensue after a natural disaster, may contribute to improving the well-being of the individual (Basoglu, Salcioglu, Livanou, Kalender & Acar, 2005).

In a study, Ironson et al. (2005) showed how dispositional optimism, less avoidant coping strategies and lower level of depression positively influence progression of the illness in patients suffering from AIDS. Although optimism is commonly believed to be a protective factor with regard to well-being and physical and psychological health Scheier, Carver, (1985). Some research has suggested that this is not always the case. Schofield et al., (2004) found that optimism did not predict lower mortality rates among lung cancer patients. Also studies concerning the immune system turned out contrasting results. Tomakowsky, Lumley, Markowitz, Frank, (2001) investigated the correlation between the "dispositional" optimism Scheier, Carver, (1985) and the "attributional" optimism Peterson C, Seligman, (1987) with the clinical and immune condition of subject affected with AIDS. The results of their research indicated that both types of optimism were associated with an improvement of the symptomatology of AIDS. Nevertheless, in the long term, high levels of optimism, in particular, of the attributional type, were associated with a significant impairment of the immune defense system.

Segerstrom, (2006) examined two hypotheses that may explain these results: the disappointment hypothesis, according to which persistent and uncontrollable stressors reduce the positive expectations that are typical of optimists and thus consequently control over the stress factors, leading to decrease in immune defense. The other is the engagement hypothesis theorizing that more optimistic individuals are more easily drawn to trying to resolve a problem while pessimists tend to let the matter drop, thus ending up more exposed to stress. As such, in cases of severe illnesses like AIDS, when associated with the elevated levels of cortisol and adrenalin that typically present when faced with stress, optimism may actually determine a decrease in the defense mechanisms of the immune system.

Positive Affectivity and Health

Emotions are biologically basic features of human functioning, and learning to regulate them constitutes a major developmental milestone (National Research Council and Institute of Medicine, 2000). Thus, patterns of emotional functioning that emerge in childhood are maintained into adulthood, and as a result child emotional functioning may provide an early indicator of adult health risk (Repetti, Taylor, & Seeman, 2002). Indeed, research is beginning to bear this out; emerging research has found that chronic high childhood distress (usually measured at age 7 or 8 years) is associated with a range of adult physical health outcomes such as obesity (Goodwin et al., 2009), number of physical ill-nesses (Kubzansky, Martin, & Buka, 2009). Support for maintaining a differentiated emotion approach is provided by the emerging research on positive emotions. One of the key theories to inform research on positive emotion and health is the Broaden-and-Build model of emotion, which identifies four positive emotion families—joy, interest, contentment, and love. While the theory was not specifically targeted to address the link between positive emotions and health, Fredrickson posited both direct effects (e.g., speeding recovery from experience of stress) and indirect effects (e.g., broadening an individual's momentary thought-action tendencies and building personal resources) that are potentially relevant for health (Fredrickson, 1998).

Generally people do not concern and need to fulfill all the materialistic requirements in order to feel cheerful, enthusiastic, and get interested in life. This general assumption focus on the philosophy, that virtually anyone is capable to experience substantial level of positive affect. Indeed, Diener and Diener (1995) demonstrated that most people regardless of their physical health state and sociocultural status experience at least moderate levels of positive affects. No doubt, some of us feel more cheerful, excited, and energetic than others. This view further raises a crucial issue: whether the long-term changes are really possible in the direction of positive affective state.

Philippe, Lecours, and Beaulieu-Pelletier (2009) stated that resilience has been frequently linked with positive affects especially under stressful and demanding situations. They raised the point that psychological processes operative in self-generation of positive emotions among resilient individuals are mostly overlooked. They further propose that emotional memories play significant role in self-generation of positive emotions. On the basis of the findings of their studies, they concluded that emotional memories networks (EMN) mediate the relationship between psychological resilience and the experience of positive emotions in the state of sadness and anxiety after controlling the pre-experimental positive mood and positive affectivity trait.

PA provides a psychological break or respite from stress, supporting continuing efforts to replenish resources depleted by stress (Lazarus, 1991; Khosla, 2006). Therefore, it is evident that PA is good for our health. Its buffering functions provide a useful antidote to the problem associated with negative emotions and ill health due to stress (Fredrickson, 2001). In a study participant experiencing PA reported having more total coping resources to deal with stress. They reported using more of problem focused coping strategies as compared to emotion focused coping strategies to cope with stress (Khosla & Hangal, 2004). PA facilitates adaptive coping and adjustment to chronic or acute stress (Folkman, 1997).

In a study it was observed that women who reported finding positive meaning in response to a traumatic event had more adaptive hormonal responses to laboratory stress induction task (Epel, McEwen & Ickovics, 1998).

Positive affect promoted coping responses which led to finding meaning in various stressful experiences (Khosla, 2006). This implies it probably has to play an active role in the prevention of adverse physiological effects of stress.

One factor that has been relatively neglected is the role of positive affect in promoting psychological resilience. Two prominent models that explain why positive affect might serve as an important factor in resilience processes guide the current research. The dynamic model of affect (Zautra, Smith, Affleck, & Tennen, 2001) and the broaden-and-build theory of positive emotions (Fredrickson, 1998) each suggest mechanisms by which positive affect promotes immediate and long-term adaptation to stress. Studies have found empirical support for both of these models (e.g. Ong, Bergeman, Bisconti, & Wallace, 2006). This study incorporates these dynamic conceptualizations to explore the role of positive affect in promoting resistance to and recovery from stress. Although positive affect may be an important factor in resilience processes, not all individuals experience positive affect during stressful times.

Smith and Baum (2003) suggested that PA may encourage restorative activities such as sleep, exercise, relaxation, vacation, and spending time in natural environments. In turn, these activities are thought to help reduce both stress appraisals and negative affective responses to stress. They also argued that positive emotions may protect persons from negative responses to stress through the release of endogenous opioids. Alternatively PA may facilitate recovery from stress-related activation.

In some studies have found that inducing amusement or contentment following a stressful or fearful stimulus results in a faster return to baseline levels of cardiovascular reactivity as does spontaneous smiling during a sadness-inducing stimulus (Fredrickson & Levenson, 1998; Fredrickson et al., 2000). In line with this, ambulatory studies have shown that HR increases last a shorter period after PA versus NA (Brosschot & Thayer, 2003) and that high happiness occurring naturally during a period of high anxiety counteracts BP increases that occur in the absence of happiness (Shapiro, Jamner, Goldstein, & Delfino, 2001).

Similarly, there is some evidence of PA's buffering the negative immune impact of ambulatory negative mood in a study showing an interaction between positive and negative mood in predicting natural killer cell activity generate psychological resources by promoting resilience, endurance, and optimism (Valdimarsdottir & Bovbjerg, 1997).

Other theorists have proposed that positive emotions do not simply buffer the effects of stress but have more direct positive effects beyond stress (Zautra et al., 2005). Although the empirical literature on positive affect and health is somewhat scattered and still limited as few studies of major health outcomes to date have been designed explicitly to examine this relationship, a promising body of evidence is beginning to emerge.

In one study, Ong and colleagues (2004) collected 98 days of daily diaries from a sample of recently bereaved older adult widows. Results of multilevel models yielded a significant Daily Stress x Daily Positive Affect interaction when predicting depressive symptoms suggesting that there was less of an increase in depressive symptoms on days of greater stress when positive affect was also higher. In other words, during times of stress, higher levels of positive affect were associated with lower negative affect (i.e. greater stress resistance).

In 2005, Pressmen and Cohen conducted a comprehensive review of the existing literature on positive affect and health and concluded that positive affect likely has a protective effect on health (Pressman & Cohen, 2005). The strongest evidence available is in relation to cardiovascular disease. Studies generally suggest that positive affect reduces risk of developing heart disease even after adjusting for known coronary risk factors as well as accounting for negative affect (Boehm & Kubzansky, 2012).

In one interesting study, positivity displayed on the faces of almost 2000 participants was judged during a structured interview (Davidson, Mostofsky, & Whang, 2010). Individuals who displayed higher levels of positive affect were at 22% reduced risk of developing heart disease over a 10-year period, after controlling for both major coronary risk factors and measures of negative affect. Additional work that has considered factors related to positive affect (e.g., optimism, emotional vitality) has also found strongly protective effects in relation to onset (as well as progression) of cardiovascular disease (Boehm & Kubzansky, 2012).

There have been a multitude of studies conducted that highlight the benefits of positive experiences and positive affect. In a review of the literature, Ryff and Singer (1998) reported that positive experience (e.g. positive life outlooks, high self-esteem, and positive affect) is associated with increases in survival time, quicker wound healing, and increases in immune functioning. In a comprehensive review of the influence of positive affect on physical health, Pressman and Cohen (2005) also cited evidence that positive affect was associated with lower morbidity, decreased symptoms and pain, and increased longevity.

Positive affect can also have an influence on various aspects of cognitive functioning. Several studies have provided evidence for a broadened scope of attention among individuals with positive emotional traits (for review, see Fredrickson, 1998). In addition, studies show that positive affect facilitates learning and mastery (for review, see Fredrickson, 1998). Isen and colleagues have provided evidence that positive affect promotes cognitive flexibility (Isen

& Daubman, 1984), facilitates creative problem solving (Isen, Johnson, Mertz, & Robinson, 1985), and promotes flexible strategy use in decision-making tasks (Isen, Rosenzweig, & Young, 1991). Ashby and colleagues (1999) propose these increases in creative problem solving may be due to increased dopamine released in the anterior cingulate that improves cognitive flexibility. The increase in dopamine is assumed to be the result of increases in positive affect. Taken together, the results of these studies highlight the beneficial role that positive affect has on physical health, psychological health, and cognitive functioning. Positive affect can serve as an important factor in two of the resilience processes previously discussed: (1) resilience as stress-resistance; and (2) resilience as recovery (Folkman & Moskowitz, 2000a; Ryff & Singer, 1998).

In separate studies, Fredrickson and colleagues (Fredrickson & Levenson, 1998; Fredrickson, Mancuso, Branigan, & Tugade, 2000; Tugade & Fredrickson, 2004) tested whether positive emotions would help to speed up cardiovascular recovery from negative emotions. In one study, participants were shown a fear-eliciting film and then randomly assigned to view a second film that elicited positive affect, negative affect, or neutrality. Results indicated that participants who viewed the positive films returned to baseline cardiovascular levels quicker than those who viewed negative and neutral films (Fredrickson & Levenson, 1998). In the second study, participants viewed a film known to elicit sadness. Interestingly, those participants who were able to spontaneously smile during the film recovered quicker, as evidenced by returning to baseline levels of cardiovascular reactivity, than those who did not smile (Fredrickson & Levenson, 1998).

Numerous studies have also shown that happy individuals (i.e. those who frequently experience positive affect) are successful in many areas, including job success, marriage, and friendship (Lyubomirsky, King, & Diener,

2005). Various reviews have considered research on subjective well-being in relation to a broad set of health outcomes, including susceptibility to infectious disease, respiratory disease, and longevity. Positive affect interacts with stress and moderates its negative effect on health (Davis et al.1998; Falk et al. 2012; Ong et al. 2006) such that the impact of stress on health is reduced when one's positive affect is high. Most have concluded that subjective well-being (and positive affect as an important sub-construct) is associated with better health, although all acknowledge wide variability in the range of outcomes and measures of positive affect, as well as the quality of the studies included in the reviews (e.g., Diener & Chan, 2011).

In present chapter we have reviewed the researches related to stress, occupational stress and health, reliance and health, optimism and health and positive affectivity and health. In the next chapter we will present the methodology related to the present study.

Chapter-III

STATEMENT OF THE PROBLEM

Globalization has led to many changes in organizational design and organizational structures, which cause stress to the employees of all types of organizational settings. The study of stress at work has become a thrust area for researchers. Stress research has paralleled the general thrust of the researchers in focusing on how to prevent and alleviate human problems and sufferings. So, stress has been studied primarily with the aim of determining how it creates problems for us and how to prevent or manage these problems. Studies in this area have investigated a number of sources and consequences of stress experienced by employees operating in different type of organizations. Health is emerging as an important factor for employees in all organization, not only in India but all over the world and it is considered as wealth.

Physical and psychological health of employees plays an important role in the smooth functioning of an organization. There are many sources of stress which affect the various domains of health of employees. Employee's physical and psychological health and wellness are adversely affected by various stress responses which include cognitive, emotional, physiological and behavioral changes. These changes are identical as a variety of feelings and reactions such as, anxiety, intense emotional and physiological arousal, depression, and frustration that may deteriorate the employees' health day by day. This kind of occupational stress results in absenteeism, higher number accidents, lower morale and greater interpersonal conflict with colleagues and supervisors. This may lead to damage mood, productivity, relationships and quality of life and well-being of employees of an organization.

The previous researches in the area of stress emphasized upon examining the physiological reactions to stress followed by an emphasis on examining coping mechanisms during stress. The same situation may be stressful to one, exiting to others, and yet some remain unaffected. This happens because of individual differences in their interpretation of event and reactions to them. These individual differences are caused by different traits, characteristics, and attributes of the focal persons. These traits or attributes may be positive or negative.

Researchers have concentrated upon the assessment of the impact of positive personal characteristics or attributes on the stress and health. Health psychologists have shown a major change of focus to the positive personal factors of health. In this study the key positive factors such as, resilience, positive affectivity, and optimism have been taken into consideration. Such positive personal or psychological factors not only add years to one's life but also add life to one's years. Positive emotion/affect has been noted to increase people's physical, cognitive and social resources, which in turn help in effective coping and living healthier (Fredericson, 2001). Positive affectivity has been found to be a good predictor of health. It has been generally found that people with high level of positive affectivity had longer life span, fewer pains and symptoms of illness (Cohen & Pressman, 2006). In a study of Yu, Zhou, and Gu (2008), found that the influence of affectivity trait or attribute on relationship between occupational stress and subjective physical health and job satisfaction. This study was conducted on 878 workers in a thermal power plant in China. The result indicates that positive affectivity was negatively and negative affectivity was positively correlated with occupational stress.

It was noted that trait resilience, which includes high level of self-esteem, personal control and optimism, appraise negative events as less stressful and revive their strength and spirit quickly (Major, et al., 1998).

Philippe, Lecours, and Beauliea-Pelletier (2009) stated that resilience frequently links with positive affect especially under stressful and demanding situations. They raised the point that psychological processes operative in self-generation of positive emotions among resilient individuals are mostly overlooked. They further proposed that emotional memories play significant role in self-regulation of positive emotions. On the basis of findings of their studies, they concluded that emotional memory networks (EMN) mediate the relationship between psychological resilience and the experience of positive emotions in the state of sadness and anxiety after controlling the pre-experimental positive mood and positive affectivity trait, respectively.

In research literature it suggests that resilience has protective nature and it helps individuals to cope with stressful events and adversity. Ong and colleagues (2006) found that trait resilience contributed to both stress resilience and recovery process. Research has consistently shown that resilient individuals have optimistic outlooks on life and are open to new experiences and have higher positive emotionality (Block & Kremen, 1996).

Further, in research literature it was noted that people expecting best and looking bright side of the things report less fatigue, fewer aches, pains and minor illness (Scheier & Carver, 1985; Scheier, Carver & Bridges, 2001). They also noted that optimists tend to have better mental and physical health and recover more quickly when they become ill. People with optimistic explanatory style tend to enjoy good health. Optimism helps in sustaining immune functions under stress (Segerstrom, et al., 1998). Optimism may significantly influence mental and physical well-being by the promotion of a healthy life style as well as by adoptive behaviors and cognitive responses, associated with greater flexibility, problem solving capacity and a more efficient elaboration of negative information (Conversano, et al., 2010). It was noted that optimists tend to experience life's difficulties with less distress than do pessimists (Scheier, et al., 2001).

Keeping in view the theoretical constructs and research findings on stress, health and positive personal attributes the present study proposed to examine the relationship of certain personal/psychological attributes with experience of stress and health status in a sample of manufacturing organizations. The study also purported to examine whether these personal attributes moderate the relationship of occupational stress and health status of the employees.

RATIONAL OF THE PROPOSED RESEARCH

In last few decades numerous studies have been conducted to examine the relationship between stress and health and its effects on employee's behavior in organizations including public and private sector employees, managerial personnel, nurses, teachers, banking sector employee, etc., but studies on supervisory level employees are relatively fewer in number.

Perhaps, with a wide range of research coverage on resilience relating it to several stress and health related psycho-social factors, there are gaps identified in the existing literature. While there is extensive coverage of children and adolescents in the resilience literature, only few studies have investigated resilience among adults and old people. Therefore, more researches are required to draw a conclusive fact about the impacts of resilience.

Although, very few studies have supported positive affectivity and optimism as a moderator of stress and health relationship, no studies are available where in resilience has been taken as moderator variable of stress and health relationship, particularly in Indian context. Keeping this in view the present study has been designed to examine the relationship between occupational stress and health as moderated by resilience, positive affectivity and optimism among supervisory level employees.

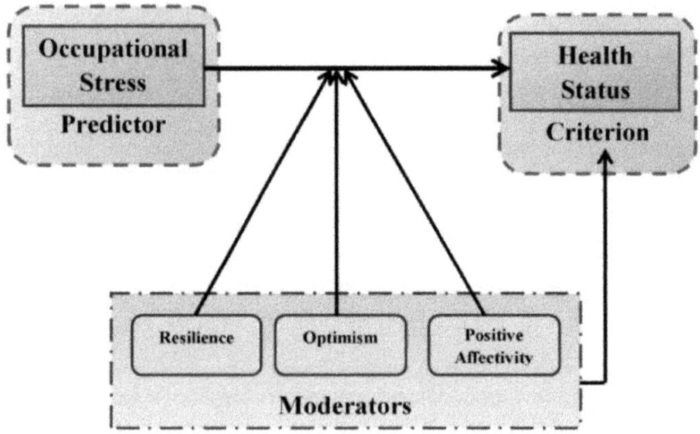

Fig 3.1 : Schematic Diagram of the Proposed Model of the Study

OBJECTIVES

The specific objectives of the present study were as follows:

1. To find out the relationship between occupational stress and health status.
2. To examine the relationship between resilience and health status.
3. To examine the relationship between optimism and health status.
4. To examine the relationship between positive affectivity and health status.
5. To examine the moderating role of resilience in the relationship between occupational stress and health status.

6. To examine the moderating role of positive affectivity in the relationship between occupational stress and health status.
7. To examine the moderating role of optimism in the relationship between occupational stress and health status.

HYPOTHESES

The following hypotheses were formulated for the present study:

1. Occupational stress would be negatively correlated with health status.
2. Resilience would be positively correlated with health status.
3. Optimism would be positively correlated with health status
4. Positive affectivity would be positively correlated with health status.
5. Resilience would moderate the relationship of occupational stress and health status.
6. Positive affectivity would moderate the relationship of occupational stress and health status.
7. Optimism would moderate the relationship of occupational stress and health status.

The present chapter was aimed to explaining the statement of the problem, rational of the present study, objectives and hypotheses. In the next chapter the methodology like, sample, design of the present study, tools of measurement, procedure and data analysis will be presented.

Chapter-IV

METHODOLOGY

The present chapter contains the description of sample on which the study was conducted, design of the study utilized in this investigation, tools of measurement, procedure of the data collection and statistical analyses.

PARTICIPANTS (SAMPLE)

"A sample is any number of persons selected to represent the population according to some rule or plan. Thus, a sample is a smaller representation of the population" (Singh, 1997). It is generally assumed that conclusions drawn on the basis of the sample may be generalized to the whole population and thereby, selection of a representative and adequately large sample is an essential prerequisite for ensuring the quality of the conducted research.

The present study was carried out on a sample of 322, but after outlier analysis finally a sample of 315 was selected for the final statistical analysis. The sample of the study comprised supervisory level employees (Age: Mean = 46.28, SD = 8.74) of manufacturing organization like, Diesel Locomotive Workshop (D.L.W), Varanasi and Railway Diesel Shed, Mughalsarai. Convenience sampling method was used in the selection of the participants for the present study. The subjects were convinced to participate in the study and they were not paid for their participation in this study.

DESIGN OF THE STUDY

The present study was an attempt to examine the relationship of stress and health status as moderated by personal attributes namely, resilience, positive affectivity and optimism among supervisory level employees of manufacturing organizations in India. The present study adopted correlational design. The occupational stress has been treated as predictor variable, health status as criterion variable and personal attributes (resilience, positive affectivity and optimism) were taken as moderator variables. We intended to examine the relationship of stress and personal variables on employee's health status. To find out the relative contribution of stress and personal attributes on health status, the stepwise multiple regression analysis has also been applied. Further, positive personal attributes was examined for their potential to moderate the relationship of stress and health status.

TOOS OF MESURMENT

Following psychometric tools were employed to assess the extent/level of different variables included in the present study.

1. Occupational Stress Index (Srivastava & Singh, 1984)

The Occupational Stress Index (O.S.I.) was used to measure the extent of stress which employees perceive arising from various constituent and conditions of their job. The scale consists of 46 items, each to be rated on the five-point scale. Out of 46 items, 28 are 'true-keyed' and rest 18 are 'false-keyed.' The items relate to almost all relevant components of the job life which cause stress in some way or the other, such as, role overload, role ambiguity, role conflict, group and political pressures, responsibility for persons, under-participation, powerlessness, poor peer relationship, intrinsic impoverishment, low status, strenuous working conditions, and unprofitability.

The reliability index as ascertained by split-half (odd-even) method and cronbach's alpha-coefficient for the scale as a whole were found to be .935 and .90, respectively. The validity of the O.S.I. was determined by computing coefficients of correlation between the scores on O.S.I. and various measures of attitudes and job behavior.

2. General Health Questionnaire (Goldberg & Hiller, 1979)

The scale measures the psychological aspect of quality of life. The scale comprises 28 items, to be rated on 4-point scale, relating to dimensions of ill-health, namely physical symptoms of ill-health, anxiety, insomnia, social dysfunction, and severe depression. High score on the scale indicates poor health. The inter-correlations between the four subscales ranged from 0.40 to 0.62, with a mean value of 0.52. The reliability of the sub-scale varies around 0.82, and mean of inter-item correlation was found to be 0.92. Validity of the scale was established by carrying out principal component analysis with varimax rotation and a forced from test or solution.

3. Resilience & optimism Scale (Srivastava, 2008)

A 5-point rating scale developed by Srivastava, (2008) was utilized to assess the extent of resilience. The scale comprises 21 items (17 true-keyed and 4 false-keyed) relating to two psychological characteristics or traits, i.e. resilience and optimism. Resilience and optimism constitute two sub-scales.

4. Positive and Negative Affect Scale (Watson, Clark, Tellegen, 1988)

The scale contains two 10-items mood scales that comprise the Positive and Negative Affect Schedules. The respondents were required to rate on 5-point scale the extent to which they experience each mood state. For the present study only positive affect schedule was used. The reliability of the scale was found to be high ranging from 0.86 to 0.90 for Positive Affects and from 0.84 to 0.87 for Negative Affect. The validity indicates that both dimensions of the scale are highly correlated with their corresponding regression-based scores in each solution with convergent correlation ranging from 0.89 to 0.95, whereas the discriminant correlations are quite low, ranging from 0.02 to 0.18.

Besides the above tests, the demographic profile of each employee was obtained as follows:

1. Name
2. Age
3. Gender
4. Qualifications
5. Profession
6. Designation
7. Marital Status
8. No. of children
9. Experience (in years)
10. Job of husband/wife

PROCEDURE OF DATA COLLATION

After selecting the tools of measurement to be used in the present investigation the necessary permission for data collection was sought from both the organizations i.e., Diesel Locomotive Work (DLW), Varanasi and Railway Diesel Shed, Mughalsarai. After receiving the required permission the tools were administered to the participants. All the participants were approached individually by the researcher and rapport was established with them. When it was found that the particular employee is convinced to participate in the study; the necessary instructions and a brief description of tests and scales along with the objectives and importance of the study were explained to the employees to insure their honest, correct and sincere responses. Afterwards all the demographic information was collected from the employees. After collecting the demographic information the Occupational Stress Index (OSI) questionnaire was given to the employee and said to read the instruction carefully before giving the responses to the items of the questionnaire. When the employee completed O.S.I.; the general heath questionnaire (GHQ) was given to the employee. Just after the completion of this questionnaire, the resilience and optimism questionnaire was administered to the employee. Finally, positive affectivity items of PANAS questionnaire was given to the employee. When the employee completed the entire questionnaire and scales the researcher thanked to the employee for their cooperation in the study.

STATISTICAL ANALYSIS OF DATA

To the raw scores obtained on different scales were entered in the computer for analyzing the data. While analyzing the data some initial or primary analysis have been done like, recoding of variables, computing variables, categorization of demographic variables, descriptive analysis, outlier analysis and scale reliability analysis. Coefficient of correlation were computed to examine the relationship between stress, positive affectivity, resilience, optimism and health status. Stepwise multiple regression analysis was run to examine the unique effects of predictor variables on criterion variables. The moderated regression analysis was done to examine the interaction of stress and positive affectivity, resilience and optimism in the prediction of health status of the participants.

Chapter-V

RESULTS

The earlier chapter dealt mainly with the concepts regarding the variables employed, a review of literature, statement of the problem and methodology adopted in the present investigation.

The present chapter embodies the results obtained from the statistical analysis of responses of the subjects on different psychometric tools. Different statistics were applied include mean, standard deviation, correlation coefficient, stepwise multiple regression analysis and moderated regression analysis to reveal the answers to the proposed research questions.

To test the hypotheses formulated for the present study that occupational stress would have positive linear relationship with physical and psychological ill health, while positive personal attributes would have inverse relationship with physical and psychological ill health of the employees in manufacturing organizations, correlational analysis was done. The results of the descriptive and correlation analysis are displayed in Table-1, 2 and 3.

Table 1 : Descriptive analysis of occupational stress, resilience, optimism, positive affectivity and ill-health and its dimensions.

Variables	Mean	Std. Deviation
Occupational Stress	123.247	20.006
Ill-Health	44.054	9.592
Somatic symptoms	11.292	3.248
Anxiety or Insomnia	10.660	3.710
Social Dysfunction	13.139	2.930
Severe Depression	8.961	2.517
Resilience	40.914	6.045
Optimism	50.231	5.118
Positive Affectivity	31.393	5.998

Note: (N=315)

The result represented in Table 1 indicates that the scores of the sample in the present study were normally distributed.

Table 2 : Coefficient of correlation between occupational stress, resilience, optimism, positive affectivity, ill-health and its dimensions.

Predictor Variables	Criterion Variables				
	Ill-Health (overall)	Somatic Symptoms	Anxiety or Insomnia	Social Dysfunction	Severe Depression
Occupational Stress	.473**	.399**	.369**	.374**	.308**
Resilience	-.506**	-.435**	-.445**	-.244**	-.429**
Optimism	-.361**	-.242**	-.249**	-.241**	-.417**
Positive Affectivity	-.047	-.034	-.015	-.003	-.115*

***p< .05, **p< .01**

The results presented in table-2 indicate that occupational stress positively and significantly relates with overall ill-health and its dimensions, namely somatic symptoms, anxiety/insomnia, social dysfunction and severe depression. Resilience negatively and significantly relates with ill-health and its four dimensions. Optimism was found to be negatively and significantly correlated with ill-health and its dimensions. Further, positive affectivity was found to be negatively but not significantly correlated with ill-health and its dimensions except severe depression.

Table 3 : Coefficients of correlation between occupational stress dimensions and ill-health dimensions.

Predictor Variables	Criterion Variables				
	Ill-Health (overall)	Somatic Symptoms	Anxiety/ Insomnia	Social Dysfunction	Severe Depression
Role Overload	.303**	.264**	.288**	.157**	.206**
Role Ambiguity	.397**	.345**	.270**	.313**	.305**
Role Conflict	.215**	.159**	.153**	.167**	.195**
Unreasonable group and Political pressures	.241**	.183**	.115*	.249**	.221**
Responsibility for persons	.075	.123*	.016	.098	-.012
Under participation	.258**	.189**	.227**	.206**	.166**
Powerlessness	.276**	.259**	.243**	.202**	.123*
Poor Peer Relations	.334**	.267**	.274**	.268**	.210**
Intrinsic Impoverishment	.286**	.227**	.203**	.289**	.160**
Low Status	.342**	.305**	.263**	.250**	.232**
Strenuous Working Conditions	.350**	.264**	.321**	.269**	.207**
Unprofitability	.198**	.173**	.165**	.201**	.055

$*p < .05$, $**p < .01$

Table 3 shows the relationship between various dimensions of occupational stress and overall ill-health and its four dimensions. The results indicate that all the dimensions of occupational stress, except responsibility for persons were found to be positively and significantly correlated with ill-health total and its dimensions. However, stress arising from responsibility for persons was found to positively correlated, though insignificantly.

Table 4 : Stepwise regression analyses using occupational stress (total & its dimensions), resilience, optimism and positive affectivity as predictors and ill-health as criterion variable.

Predictor Variables	β	R	R^2	Adjusted R^2	ΔR^2	F
Resilience	-.506	.506	.256	.254	.256	107.901***
Occupational Stress	.336	.596	.355	.351	.098	85.800***
Role Conflict	-.143	.605	.366	.360	.011	59.866***
Intrinsic Impoverishment	-.161	.615	.378	.370	.012	47.061***
Under participation	-.140	.623	.388	.378	.010	39.230***
Optimism	-.118	.630	.397	.385	.009	33.795***

Criterion Variable: ill-Health *p< .05, **p< .01, ***p< .001

Stepwise regression analysis was applied to find out the relative contribution of various personal attributes, occupational stress and its dimensions to total variance in mental and physical ill-health symptoms. The results recorded in Table 4 indicate that resilience accounted for a maximum variance (i.e. 25.6%) in the symptoms of ill-health and it emerge as a preventive predictor of ill-health (β = - 0.506, $p < 0.001$). If the resilience is high, ill-health symptoms of ill-health decrease. Occupational stress accounted for 9.8% variance and its dimensions like, role conflict (1.1%), intrinsic impoverishment (1.2%) and under participation (1.0%) indicated causing significant variance in ill-health symptoms. Optimism was also found contribute 0.9% to the variance in ill-health symptoms of the employees.

Table 5 : Stepwise regression analyses using occupational stress (total & its dimensions), resilience, optimism and positive affectivity as predictors and somatic symptoms as criterion variable.

Predictor Variables	β	R	R^2	Adjusted R^2	ΔR^2	F
Resilience	-0.435	0.435	0.189	0.186	0.189	72.931***
Occupational Stress	0.280	0.508	0.258	0.253	0.069	54.140***
Role Conflict	-0.160	0.521	0.272	0.265	0.014	38.688***
Under participation	-0.171	0.536	0.288	0.278	0.016	31.277***
Intrinsic Impoverishment	-0.177	0.549	0.302	0.290	0.014	26.700***
Powerlessness	0.181	0.562	0.316	0.303	0.014	23.709***
Role Overload	-0.147	0.570	0.325	0.309	0.009	21.101***

Criterion Variable: somatic symptoms *p< .05, **p< .01, ***p< .001

Result presented in Table 5 shows that resilience has emerged as a most dominant predictor of somatic symptoms (β = -0.160, p < 0.001). Other effective predictors emerged in regression analysis were occupational stress (β = - 0.280, P < 0.001), role conflict (β = - 0.160, p < 0.001), under participation (β = - 0.171, p < 0.001), intrinsic imporishment (β = - 0.177, p < 0.001), powerlessness (β = 0.181, p < 0.001) and role overload (β = - 0.147, p < 0.001). The results suggest that resilience accounted for 18.9% of total variance, followed by occupational stress (6.9%), role conflict (1.4%), under participation (1.6%), intrinsic impoverishment (1.4%), powerlessness (1.4%) and role overload (0.9%) in the somatic symptoms.

Table 6 : Stepwise regression analyses using occupational stress (total & its dimensions), resilience, optimism and positive affectivity as predictors and anxiety or insomnia as criterion variable.

Predictor Variables	β	R	R^2	Adjusted R^2	ΔR^2	F
Resilience	-0.445	0.445	0.198	0.196	0.198	77.311***
Occupational Stress	0.242	0.499	0.249	0.244	0.051	51.761***
Intrinsic Impoverishment	-0.157	0.510	0.260	0.253	0.011	36.511***
Role Conflict	-0.149	0.522	0.273	0.263	0.012	29.035***

Criterion Variable: anxiety or insomnia, *p< .05, **p< .01, ***p< .001

The results depicted in Table 6 make it apparent that resilience was predominant predictor (β= -0.445, $p < 0.001$) of anxiety or insomnia and it predicted 19.8% of the total variance in symptoms of anxiety or insomnia. Occupational stress (β = 0.242, $p < 0.001$) explained 5.1% of variance, intrinsic imporishment (β = - 0.157, $p < 0.001$) explained 1.1% of variance and role conflict (β = - 0.149, $p < 0.001$) explained 1.2% of variance in anxiety or insomnia.

Table 7 : Stepwise regression analyses using occupational stress (total & its dimensions), resilience, optimism and positive affectivity as predictors and social dysfunction as criterion variable.

Predictor Variables	β	R	R^2	Adjusted R^2	ΔR^2	F
Occupational Stress	0.374	0.374	0.140	0.137	0.140	51.023***
Optimism	-0.164	0.407	0.166	0.160	0.026	31.003***
Role Conflict	-0.156	0.423	0.179	0.171	0.013	22.638***
Under participation	-0.139	0.435	0.189	0.179	0.010	18.111***
Role Overload	-0.169	0.452	0.205	0.192	0.015	15.887***

Criterion Variable: social dysfunction, *p< .05, **p< .01, ***p< .001

The result presented in the Table 7 indicates that occupational stress has emerged as a dominant predictor (β = 0.374, p < 0.001) of social dysfunction and explain 14.0% of the total variance in it. Other effective predictors emerged in the regression analysis were optimism (β = - 0.164, p < 0.001) explained 2.6% of variance, role conflict (β = - 0.156, p < 0.001) explained 1.3% of variance, under participation (β = - 0.139, p < 0.001) explained 1.0% of variance and role overload (β = - 0.169, p < 0.001) explained 1.5% of variance in social dysfunction.

Table 8 : Stepwise regression analyses using occupational stress (total & its dimensions), resilience, optimism and positive affectivity as predictors and severe depression as criterion variable.

Predictor Variables	β	R	R^2	Adjusted R^2	ΔR^2	F
Resilience	-0.429	0.429	0.184	0.181	0.184	70.551***
Role Ambiguity	0.214	0.476	0.227	0.222	0.043	45.811***
Optimism	-0.248	0.517	0.267	0.260	0.040	37.756***

Criterion Variable: Severe depression, *p< .05, **p< .01, ***p< .001

Further, the result of regression Table 8 revealed that resilience has emerged as a best predictor (β = - 0.429, p < 0.001) of severe depression and it explain 18.4% of the total variance in it. Role ambiguity (β = 0.214, p < 0.001) explains 4.3% of variance and optimism (β = - 0.248, p < 0.001) accounted 4.0% of variance in severe depression.

The above mentioned section demonstrate that stress and health correlated significantly in the expected direction that is; high stress was found to be associated with poor health and greater complaints of physical and mental/psychological health problems. Given the relationship between stress and health, an attempt was made to explore that how and to what extent positive personal attributes moderate this relationship. It has been hypothesized in present research that, positive personal attributes (Resilience, Positive affectivity and Optimism) are likely to moderate this relationship. This speculation is based on the earlier and present research findings that positive personal attributes correlates significantly with both stress and health.

To test the hypotheses of moderation the statistical technique of moderated regression analysis was used. Positive personal attributes were examined for the probable moderated regression analyses have been presented which indicated a significant moderation effect.

To examine the moderating role of resilience in stress-health relationship moderated regression analysis was performed. Various dimensions of ill-health (Anxiety, Depression, Somatic Symptoms and Social Dysfunction) as well as ill-health (total) were entered as dependent variable, predictor variable (Occupational Stress) was enter in the first step, moderator variable (Resilience) enter in the second step of the model and cross product of occupational stress and resilience were entered in the third step of the model. The obtained result has been presented in Table 9.

Table 9 : Moderated regression analyses of resilience as a moderator of the relationship between occupational stress and ill-health.

Variables	R	R^2	Adjusted R^2	ΔR^2	ΔF	Sig
Occupational Stress	.473	.224	.222	.224	90.341	.000
Resilience	.596	.355	.351	.131	63.282	.000
O. Stress X Resilience	.627	.393	.387	.038	19.471	.000

Criterion Variable: ill-Health

The result presented in Table 9 indicate that R square value for the occupational stress explains 22.4% of variance in ill-health total, resilience explains 35.5% of variance in ill-health and occupational stress and resilience together explains the 39.3% of variance in ill-health total. Further R square change for the occupational stress accounted for 22.4% of variance, resilience accounted for 13.1% of variance. When interaction term is added together the predictor and moderator variables, R square change became 0.038 and explain additionally 3.8% of variance in ill-health. This change is highly significant ($F = 19.471$, $p < 0.001$). This interaction result shows that resilience significantly moderates the adverse effect of occupational stress on health of the employees. This moderation effect is shown in the graph below in Figure 5.1.

Figure 5.1 : Graph showing the interaction/ moderating effect of resilience in the relationship between occupational stress and ill-health.

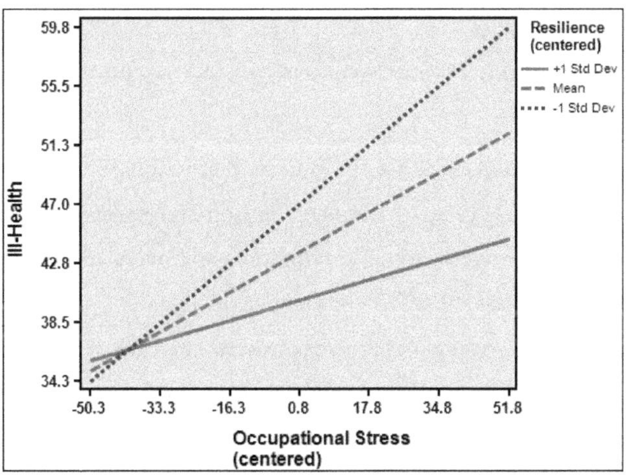

From the interaction graph it is evident that under low occupational stress condition, different levels of resilience do not have any significant effect on ill-health. However, under high occupational stress condition, the presence of resilience would lower the ill-health symptoms and enhance good health of the employees. It can be also said that when resilience is low, the effect of occupational stress on ill-health is increases and health became poor. However, when resilience is high, the effect of stress on ill-health is reduced and the relationship between occupational stress and ill-health is weaker. Employees with high resilience show lower ill-health symptoms in stressful situations or in other words have better health even in varying stressful situation than lower resilience counterparts.

Table 10 : Moderated regression analyses of resilience as a moderator of the relationship between Occupational Stress and Somatic Symptoms.

Variables	R	R^2	Adjusted R^2	ΔR^2	ΔF	Sig
Occupational Stress	.399	.160	.157	.160	59.413	.000
Resilience	.508	.258	.253	.098	41.230	.000
O. Stress X Resilience	.544	.296	.289	.038	16.732	.000

Criterion Variable: Somatic Symptoms, *p< .05, **p< .01, ***p< .001

The result of Table 10 indicate that R square value for the occupational stress explains 16% of variance in somatic symptoms, resilience explains 25.8% of variance in somatic symptoms and occupational stress and resilience together explains the 29.6% of variance in somatic symptoms. Further R square change for the occupational stress is accounted for 16% of variance, resilience accounted 9.8% of variance and when interaction term is added together the predictor and moderator variables, R square change became 0.038 and explain additionally 3.8% of variance in somatic symptoms. This change is highly significant ($F= 16.732$, $p < 0.001$). This interaction result shows that the presumed moderator resilience significantly moderates the adverse effect of occupational stress on somatic symptoms of ill-health of employees. This moderation effect is shown in Figure 5.2.

Figure 5.2 : Graph showing the interaction/moderating effect of resilience in the relationship between occupational stress and somatic symptoms of ill-health.

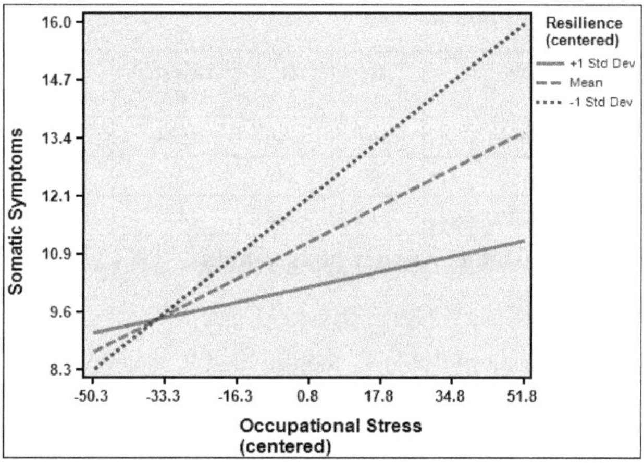

From the interaction graph it is clear that the positive relationship between occupational stress and somatic symptoms of ill-health is getting weaker when resilience is concerned. Employees with high resilience show lower somatic symptoms of health in stressful situation than low resilience counterparts. In other words we can say according to interaction graph that when occupational stress is high, somatic symptoms of health is also high and resilience is low and when resilience is high it reduces the effect of occupational stress on somatic symptoms of ill-health and weaken their relationship, it means that resilience moderate the relationship between occupational stress and somatic symptoms of ill-health.

Table 11 : Moderated regression analyses of resilience as a moderator of the relationship between Occupational Stress and Anxiety or Insomnia.

Variables	R	R^2	Adjusted R^2	ΔR^2	ΔF	Sig
Occupational Stress	.369	.136	.134	.136	49.456	.000
Resilience	.499	.249	.244	.113	46.826	.000
O. Stress X Resilience	.512	.262	.255	.013	5.411	.021

Criterion Variable: Anxiety or Insomnia

The result of Table 11 indicate that R square value for the occupational stress explains 13.6% of variance in anxiety or insomnia, resilience explains 24.9% of variance in anxiety or insomnia and occupational stress and resilience together explains the 26.2% of variance in anxiety or insomnia. Further R square change for the occupational stress accounted for 13.6% of variance, resilience accounted for 11.3% of variance and when interaction term is added together the predictor and moderator variables, R square change became 0.013 and explain additional only 1.3% of variance in anxiety or insomnia. This change is significant ($F= 5.411$, $p < 0.05$). This interaction result shows that the presumed moderator resilience markedly moderates the effect of occupational stress on anxiety or insomnia symptoms of ill-health. This moderating effect is show in the graph below in Figure 5.3.

Figure 5.3 : Graph showing the interaction/moderating effect of resilience in the relationship between occupational stress and anxiety/insomnia symptoms of ill-health.

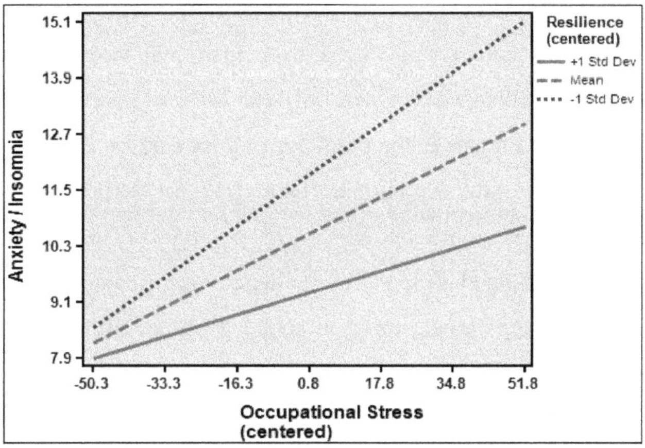

It is evident from the interaction graph (Figure 5.3) that under low occupational stress condition, different levels of resilience do not have any significant effect on anxiety / insomnia. However, under high occupational stress condition, the high resilient employees would show lower or less anxiety /insomnia symptoms of ill-health. So it can say that resilience moderate the occupational stress and anxiety /insomnia relationship.

Table 12 : Moderated regression analyses of resilience as a moderator of the relationship between Occupational Stress and Social Dysfunction.

Variables	R	R^2	Adjusted R^2	ΔR^2	ΔF	Sig
Occupational Stress	.374	.140	.137	.140	51.023	.000
Resilience	.393	.154	.149	.014	5.151	.024
O. Stress X Resilience	.406	.165	.157	.011	3.995	.046

Criterion Variable: Social Dysfunction

The result shown on Table 12 indicate that R square value for the occupational stress explains 14% of variance in social dysfunction, resilience explains 15.4% of variance in social dysfunction and occupational stress and resilience together explains the 16.5% of variance in social dysfunction. Further R square change for the occupational stress accounted for 14% of variance, resilience accounted only for 1.4% of variance and when interaction term is added together the predictor and moderator variables, R square change became 0.011 and explain additional 1.1% of variance in social dysfunction. This change is significant ($F= 3.995$, $p < 0.05$). This interaction result shows that the presumed moderator resilience significantly moderates the adverse effect of occupational stress on social dysfunction. This moderating effect is show in the graph below in Figure 5.4.

Figure 5.4 : Graph showing the interaction / moderating effect of resilience in the relationship between occupational stress and social dysfunction symptoms of ill-health.

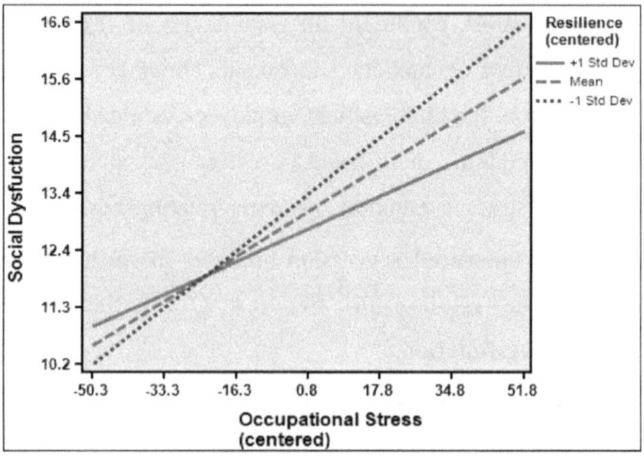

Figure 5.4 shows that under low stress condition, different levels of resilience do not have any significant effect on social dysfunction symptoms of ill-health. However, under high stress condition, the presence of resilience would lower social dysfunction. It means that resilience moderate the occupational stress and social dysfunction relationship.

Table 13 : Moderated regression analyses of resilience as a moderator of the relationship between Occupational Stress and Severe Depression.

Variables	R	R^2	Adjusted R^2	ΔR^2	ΔF	Sig
Occupational Stress	.308	.095	.092	.095	32.726	.000
Resilience	.460	.212	.206	.117	46.245	.000
O. Stress X Resilience	.503	.253	.246	.042	17.347	.000

Criterion Variable: Severe Depression

The result of Table 13 indicate that R square value for the occupational stress explains 9.5% of variance in severe depression, resilience explains 21.2% of variance in severe depression and occupational stress and resilience together explain 25.3% of variance in severe depression. Further R square change for the occupational stress accounted for 9.5% of variance, resilience accounted for 11.7% of variance and when interaction term is added together with the predictor and moderator variables, R square change became 0.042 and explains additional 4.2% of variance in severe depression. This change is highly significant F= 17.347, $p < 0.001$. This interaction result shows that the presumed moderator resilience significantly moderates the adverse effect of occupational stress on severe depression. This moderating effect is show in the graph below in Figure 5.5.

Figure 5.5 : Graph showing the interaction / moderating effect of resilience in the relationship between occupational stress and severe depression symptoms of ill-health.

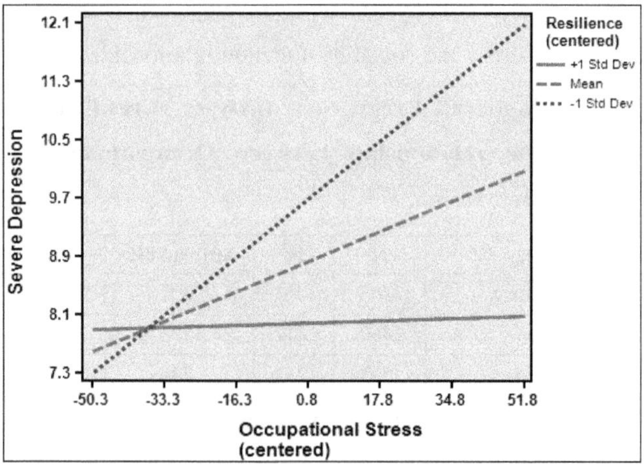

From the interaction graph (Figure 5.5) clear that under low occupational stress condition, different levels of resilience do not have any significant effect on severe depression symptoms of ill-health. However, under high occupational stress condition, the presence of resilience would lower the symptoms of severe depression and enhancing the better health of employees.

Table 14 : Moderated regression analyses of Optimism as a moderator of the relationship between Occupational Stress and ill-health.

Variables	R	R^2	Adjusted R^2	ΔR^2	ΔF	Sig
Occupational Stress	.473	.224	.222	.224	90.341	.000
Optimism	.562	.316	.312	.092	42.051	.000
O. Stress X Optimism	.591	.350	.344	.034	16.109	.000

Criterion Variable: ill-Health

The result of Table 14 indicate that R square value for the occupational stress explains 22.4% of variance in ill-health total, optimism explains 31.6% of variance in ill-health and occupational stress and optimism together explain 35% of variance in ill-health total. Further R square change for the occupational stress accounted for 22.4% of variance, optimism accounted for 9.2% of variance and when interaction term is added together with the predictor and moderator variables, R square change became 0. 034 and explains additional 3.4% of variance in ill-health total. This change is highly significant (F= 16.109, $p < 0.001$). This interaction result shows that the presumed moderator optimism significantly moderate the adverse effect of occupational stress on the ill-health. This moderating effect is show in the graph below in Figure 5.6.

Figure 5.6 : Graph showing the interaction / moderating effect of optimism in the relationship between occupational stress and ill-health.

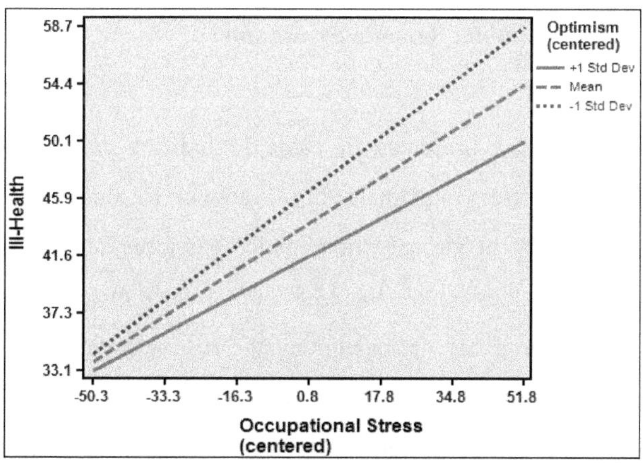

From the interaction graph (Figure 5.6) it is evident that the positive relationship between occupational stress and ill-health is getting weaker when optimism is concerned. That indicates optimism buffer / moderate the negative impact of occupational stress on health by changing the direction of the relationship between these two (PV and CV). According to graph it is evident that employees with high optimism shows lower poor health symptoms in stressful situation or in varing stressful situation than lower optimistic counterparts. The outcome of this interaction is that optimism serve as a moderator of the relationship between occupational stress and ill-health of employees.

Table 15 : Moderated regression analyses of Optimism as a moderator of the relationship between Occupational Stress and Somatic Symptoms.

Variables	R	R^2	Adjusted R^2	ΔR^2	ΔF	Sig
Occupational Stress	.399	.160	.157	.160	59.413	.000
Optimism	.466	.217	.212	.057	22.906	.000
O. Stress X Optimism	.504	.255	.247	.037	15.635	.000

Criterion Variable: Somatic Symptoms

The result presented in Table 15 indicate that R square value for the occupational stress explains 16% of variance in somatic symptoms, optimism explains 21.7% of variance in somatic symptoms and occupational stress and optimism together explain the 25.5% of variance in somatic symptoms. Further R square change for the occupational stress accounted for 16% of variance, optimism accounted for 5.7% of variance and when interaction term is added together with the predictor and moderator variables, R square change became 0. 037 and explain additional 3.7% of variance in somatic symptoms. This change is highly significant ($F= 15.635$, $p < 0.001$). This interaction result shows that the presumed moderator optimism significantly moderates the effect of occupational stress on somatic symptoms. It can be said that optimism is found to be the important moderator of the relationship between occupational stress and somatic symptoms. This moderating effect is show in the graph below in Figure 5.7.

Figure 5.7 : Graph showing the interaction / moderating effect of optimism in the relationship between occupational stress and somatic symptoms of ill-health.

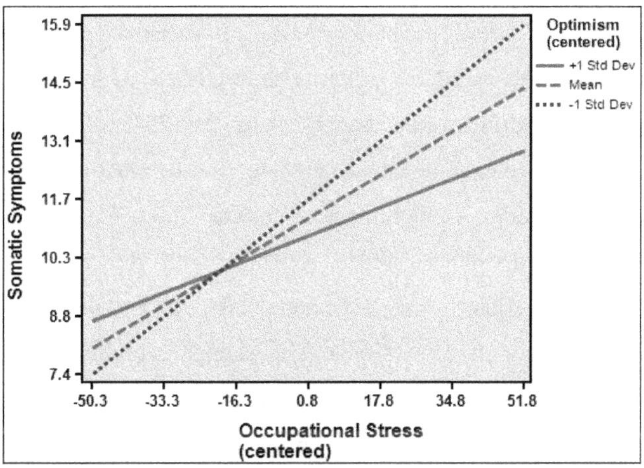

The interaction graph depicted in Figure 5.7 make it apparent that under low occupational stress condition, different levels of optimism do not have any significant effect on somatic symptoms of ill-health. However, under high occupational stress condition, the presence of high optimism would lower somatic symptoms thereby enhancing better health of employees.

Table 16 : Moderated regression analyses of Optimism as a moderator of the relationship between Occupational Stress and Anxiety or Insomnia.

Variables	R	R^2	Adjusted R^2	ΔR^2	ΔF	Sig
Occupational Stress	.369	.136	.134	.136	49.456	.000
Optimism	.476	.227	.222	.090	36.386	.000
O. Stress X Optimism	.500	.250	.243	.023	9.654	.002

Criterion Variable: Anxiety or Insomnia

The result presented in Table 16 indicate that R square value for the occupational stress explains 13.6% of variance in anxiety or insomnia, optimism explains 22.7% of variance in anxiety or insomnia and occupational stress and optimism together explains the 25% of variance in anxiety or insomnia. Further R square change for the occupational stress accounted for 13.6% of variance, optimism accounted for 9% of variance and when interaction variable is added together with the predictor and moderator variables, R square change became 0.023 and explains additional 2.3% of variance in anxiety or insomnia. This change is highly significant ($F= 9.654$, $p < 0.001$). This interaction result shows that the presumed moderator optimism markedly moderates the effect of predictor (occupational stress) on the criterion variable (anxiety or insomnia). It can be said that optimism is found to be the significant moderator of the relationship between occupational stress and anxiety or insomnia. This moderating effect is show in the graph below in Figure 5.8.

Figure 5.8 : Graph showing the interaction / moderating effect of optimism in the relationship between occupational stress and anxiety / insomnia symptoms of ill-health.

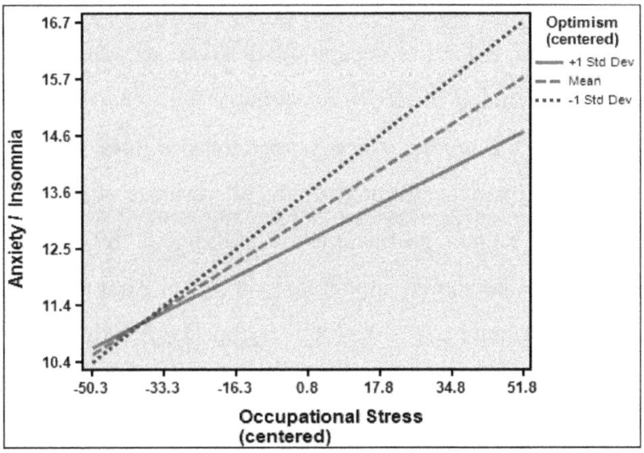

The interaction graph of Figure 5.8 again indicates that under low occupational stress condition, different levels of optimism do not have any significant effect on anxiety / insomnia symptoms of ill-health. However, under high occupational stress condition, the presence of optimism would lower the symptoms of anxiety /insomnia of employees.

Table 17 : Moderated regression analyses of Optimism as a moderator of the relationship between Occupational Stress and Social Dysfunction.

Variables	R	R^2	Adjusted R^2	ΔR^2	ΔF	Sig
Occupational Stress	.374	.140	.137	.140	51.023	.000
Optimism	.407	.166	.160	.026	9.583	.002
O. Stress X Optimism	.413	.171	.163	.005	1.898	.169

Criterion Variable: Social Dysfunction

The result presented in Table 17 indicate that R square value for the occupational stress explains 14% of variance in social dysfunction, optimism explains 16.6% of variance in social dysfunction and occupational stress and optimism together explain the 17.1% of variance in social dysfunction. Further R square change for the occupational stress accounted for 14% of variance, optimism accounted for 2.6% of variance and when interaction term is added together with the predictor and moderator variables, R square change became 0.005 and explains additional 0.5% of variance in social dysfunction. This change is not found significant ($F= 1.898$, $p < 0.169$). So the interaction result clear that the presumed moderator optimism slightly moderate the adverse effect of occupational stress on social dysfunction, but it is not found significant moderator of the relationship between occupational stress and social dysfunction. This is show in the graph below in Figure 5.9.

Figure 5.9 : Graph showing the interaction / moderating effect of optimism in the relationship between occupational stress and social dysfunction symptoms of ill-health.

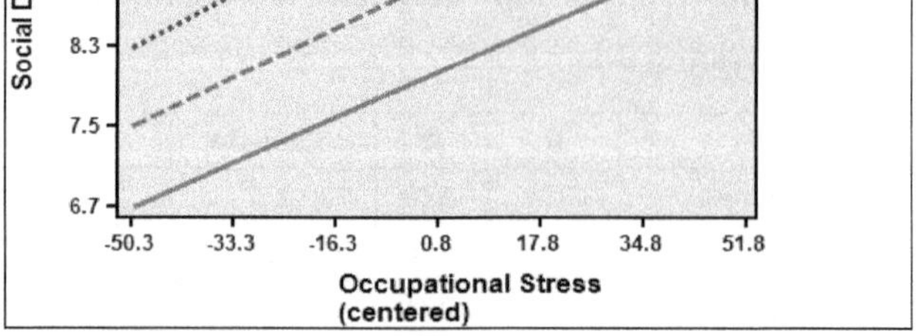

The interaction graph of Figure 5.9 shows that lower levels of optimism do not have any effect on social dysfunction but high levels of optimism lower the effect of occupational stress on symptoms of social dysfuction of the employees but there is no interaction found in this graph. It means that optimism is not found as a significant moderator between the relationship of occupational stress and social dysfuction.

Table 18 : Moderated regression analyses of Optimism as a moderator of the relationship between Occupational Stress and Severe Depression.

Variables	R	R^2	Adjusted R^2	ΔR^2	ΔF	Sig
Occupational Stress	.308	.095	.092	.095	32.726	.000
Optimism	.404	.163	.157	.068	25.405	.000
O. Stress X Optimism	.441	.195	.187	.032	12.241	.001

Criterion Variable: Severe Depression

The result depicted in Table 18 indicate that R square value for the occupational stress explains 9.5% of variance in severe depression, optimism explains 16.3% of variance in severe depression and occupational stress and optimism together explain the 19.5% of variance in severe depression. Further R square change for the occupational stress accounted for 9.5% of variance, optimism accounted for 6.8% of variance and when interaction term is added together with the predictor and moderator variables, R square change became 0.032 and explains additional 3.2% of variance in severe depression. This change is highly significant ($F= 12.241$, $p < 0.001$). This interaction result shows that the presumed moderator optimism markedly moderates the effect of occupational stress on severe depression. This moderating effect is show in the graph below in Figure 5.10.

Figure 5.10 : Graph showing the interaction / moderating effect of optimism in the relationship between occupational stress and severe depression symptoms of ill-health.

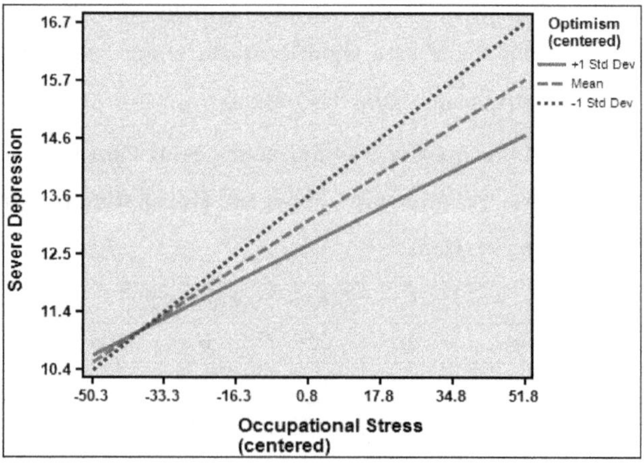

From the interaction graph (Figure 5.10) it is evident that under low occupational stress condition, different levels of optimism do not have any significant effect on severe depression symptoms of ill-health. However, under high occupational stress condition, the presence of optimism would lower the symptoms of severe depression. It means that optimism is a significant moderator of the relationship between occupational stress and severe depression symptoms of ill-health.

Table 19 : Moderated regression analyses of Positive Affectivity as a moderator of the relationship between Occupational Stress and ill-health.

Variables	R	R^2	Adjusted R^2	ΔR^2	ΔF	Sig
Occupational Stress	.473	.224	.222	.224	90.341	.000
Positive Affectivity	.475	.226	.221	.002	.819	.366
O. Stress X PA	.503	.253	.245	.027	11.035	.001

Criterion Variable: ill-Health

The result presented in Table 19 indicate that R square value for the occupational stress explains 22.4% of variance in ill-health total, positive affectivity explains 22.6% of variance in ill-health and occupational stress and positive affectivity together explains 25.3% of variance in ill-health total. Further R square change for the occupational stress accounted for 22.4% of variance, positive affectivity accounted only for 0.2% of variance and when interaction variable is added together with the predictor and moderator variables, R square change became 0.027 and explains additional 2.7% of variance in ill-health total. This change is highly significant (F= 11.035, p < 0.001). This interaction result shows that the presumed moderator positive affectivity significantly moderates the effect of occupational stress on ill-health. This moderating effect is show in the graph below in Figure 5.11.

Figure 5.11 : Graph showing the interaction / moderating effect of positive affectivity in the relationship between occupational stress and ill-health total.

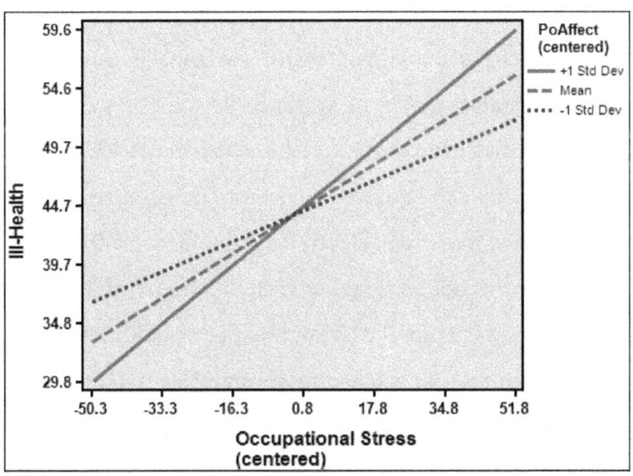

The interaction graph of Figure 5.11 is shows that under low stress condition, the different levels of positive affectivity does not aggravates the ill effects of occupational stress on ill-health. However, under high occupational stress condition positive affectivity aggravates the ill effects of occupational stress on ill-health of the employees. Hence we see that positive affectivity is a negative moderator of ill-health under high occupational stress condition.

Table 20 : Moderated regression analyses of Positive Affectivity as a moderator of the relationship between Occupational Stress and Somatic Symptoms.

Variables	R	R^2	Adjusted R^2	ΔR^2	ΔF	Sig
Occupational Stress	.399	.160	.157	.160	59.413	.000
Positive Affectivity	.402	.161	.156	.002	.709	.400
O. Stress X PA	.416	.173	.165	.012	4.452	.036

Criterion Variable: Somatic Symptoms

The result presented in Table 20 indicate that R square value for the occupational stress explains 16% of variance in somatic symptoms, positive affectivity explains 16.1% of variance in somatic symptoms and occupational stress and positive affectivity together explain the 17.3% of variance in somatic symptoms. Further R square change for the occupational stress accounted for 16% of variance, positive affectivity accounted for 0.2% of variance and when interaction term is added together with the predictor and moderator variables, R square change became 0.012 and explains additional 1.2% of variance in somatic symptoms. This change is significant ($F= 4.452$, $p < 0.05$). This interaction result shows that the presumed moderator positive affectivity moderate the adverse effect of occupational stress on somatic symptoms of ill-health of the employees. This moderation effect is shown in the graph below in figure 5.12.

Figure 5.12 : Graph showing the interaction / moderating effect of positive affectivity in the relationship between occupational stress and somatic symptoms of ill-health.

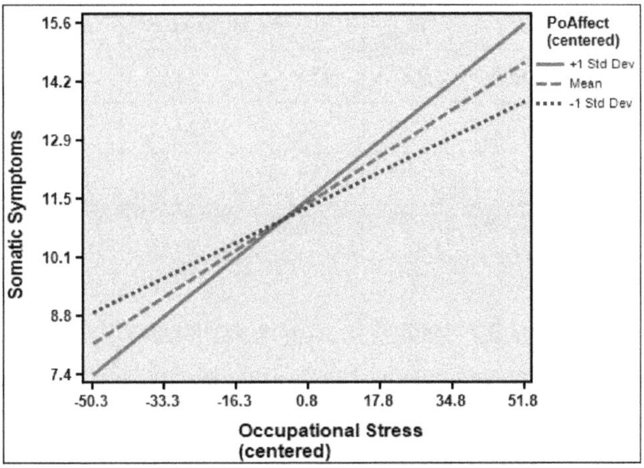

The interaction graph of Figure 5.12 is shows that under low stress condition, the different levels of positive affectivity does not aggravates the ill effects of occupational stress on somatic symptoms. However, under high occupational stress condition positive affectivity aggravates the ill effects of occupational stress on somatic symptoms of the employees. Hence we see that positive affectivity is a negative moderator of somatic symptoms under high occupational stress condition.

Table 21 : Moderated regression analyses of Positive Affectivity as a moderator of the relationship between Occupational Stress and Anxiety or Insomnia.

Variables	R	R^2	Adjusted R^2	ΔR^2	ΔF	Sig
Occupational Stress	.369	.136	.134	.136	49.456	.000
Positive Affectivity	.374	.140	.134	.003	1.173	.280
O. Stress X PA	.397	.157	.149	.018	6.499	.011

Criterion Variable: Anxiety or Insomnia

The result presented in Table 21 indicate that R square value for the occupational stress explains 13.6% of variance in anxiety or insomnia, positive affectivity explains 14% of variance in anxiety or insomnia and occupational stress and positive affectivity together explain the 15.7% of variance in anxiety or insomnia. Further R square change for the occupational stress accounted for 13.6% of variance, positive affectivity accounted for 0.3% of variance and when interaction term is added together with the predictor and moderator variables, R square change became 0.018 and explains additional 1.8% of variance in anxiety or insomnia. This change is significant ($F= 6.499$, $p < 0.05$). This interaction result shows that the presumed moderator positive affectivity significantly moderates the effect of occupational stress on anxiety or insomnia. This moderating effect is show in the graph below in Figure 5.13.

Figure 5.13 : Graph showing the interaction / moderating effect of positive affectivity in the relationship between occupational stress and anxiety / insomnia symptoms of ill-health.

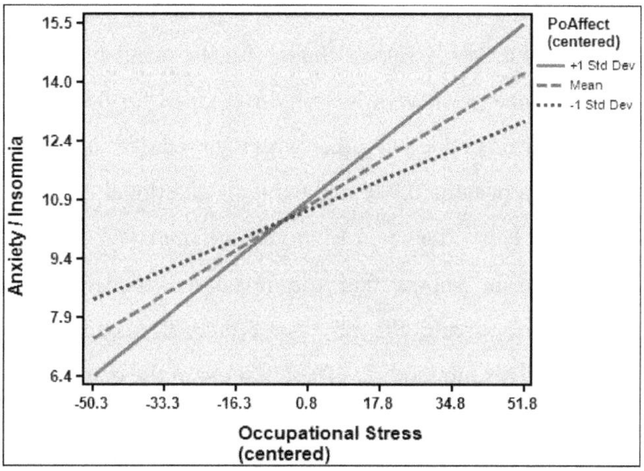

The interaction graph of Figure 5.13 is shows that under low stress condition, the different levels of positive affectivity does not aggravates the ill effects of occupational stress on anxiety / insomnia symptoms of ill-health. However, under high occupational stress condition positive affectivity aggravates the ill effects of occupational stress on anxiety / insomnia of the employees. Hence we see that positive affectivity is a negative moderator of anxiety / insomnia under high occupational stress condition.

Table 22 : Moderated regression analyses of Positive Affectivity as a moderator of the relationship between Occupational Stress and Social Dysfunction.

Variables	R	R^2	Adjusted R^2	ΔR^2	ΔF	Sig
Occupational Stress	.374	.140	.137	.140	51.023	.000
Positive Affectivity	.382	.146	.141	.006	2.128	.146
O. Stress X PA	.415	.172	.164	.026	9.818	.002

Criterion Variable: Social Dysfunction

The result presented in Table 22 indicate that R square value for the occupational stress explains 14% of variance in social dysfunction, positive affectivity explains 14.6% of variance in social dysfunction and occupational stress and positive affectivity together explain the 17.2% of variance in social dysfunction. Further R square change for the occupational stress accounted for 14% of variance, positive affectivity accounted for 0.6% of variance and when interaction term is added together with the predictor and moderator variables, R square change became 0.026 and explains additional 2.6% of variance in social dysfunction. This change is highly significant ($F= 9.818$, $p < 0.001$). This interaction result shows that the presumed moderator positive affectivity significantly moderate the adverse effect of occupational stress on social dysfunction. This moderating effect is show in the graph below in Figure 5.14.

Figure 5.14 : Graph showing the interaction / moderating effect of positive affectivity in the relationship between occupational stress and social dysfunction symptoms of ill-health.

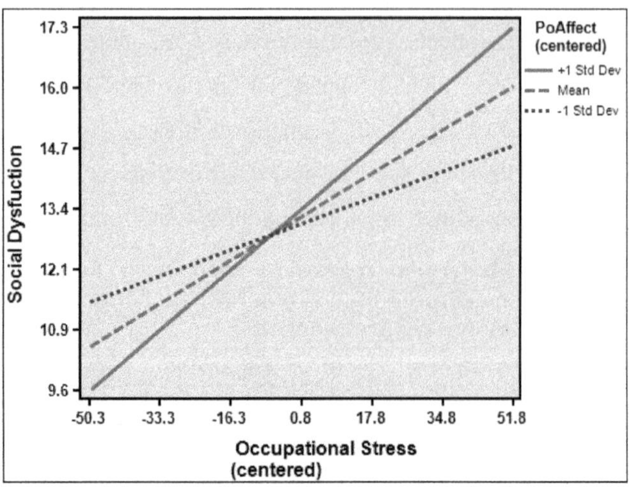

The interaction graph of Figure 5.14 is shows that under low stress condition, the different levels of positive affectivity does not aggravates the ill effects of occupational stress on social dysfunction. However, under high occupational stress condition positive affectivity aggravates the ill effects of occupational stress on social dysfunction of the employees. Hence we see that positive affectivity is a negative moderator of social dysfunction under high occupational stress condition.

Table 23 : Moderated regression analyses of Positive Affectivity as a moderator of the relationship between Occupational Stress and Severe Depression.

Variables	R	R^2	Adjusted R^2	ΔR^2	ΔF	Sig
Occupational Stress	.308	.095	.092	.095	32.726	.000
Positive Affectivity	.313	.098	.092	.003	1.135	.288
O. Stress X PA	.327	.107	.099	.009	3.236	.073

Criterion Variable: Severe Depression

The result of table-23 indicate that R square value for the occupational stress explains 9.5% of variance in severe depression, positive affectivity explains 9.8% of variance in severe depression and occupational stress and positive affectivity together explain the 10.7% of variance in severe depression. Further R square change for the occupational stress accounted for 9.5% of variance, positive affectivity accounted only for 0.3% of variance and when interaction term is added together with the predictor and moderator variables, R square change became 0.009 and explains additional 0.9% of variance in severe depression. This change is not significant ($F= 3.236$, $p < 0.073$). This interaction result shows that the presumed moderator positive affectivity dose not moderate the adverse effect of occupational stress on severe depression. It may be concluded that positive affectivity is not a significant moderator of the relationship between occupational stress and severe depression. This is show in the graph below in Figure 5.15.

Figure 5.15 : Graph showing the interaction / moderating effect of positive affectivity in the relationship between occupational stress and severe depression symptoms of ill-health.

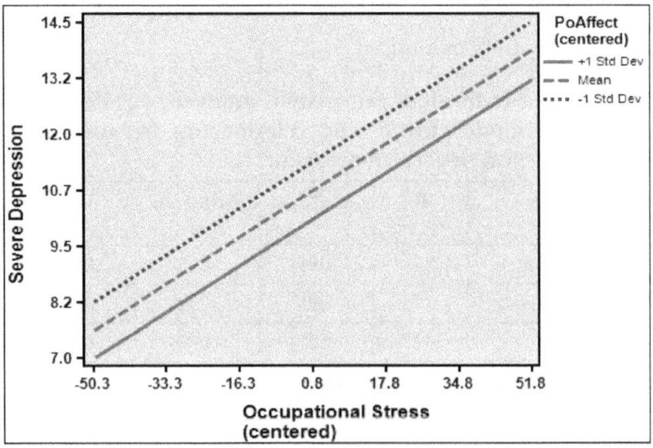

The interaction graph of Figure 5.15 shows that lower levels of positive affectivity do not have any effect on severe depression but high levels of positive affectivity lower the effect of occupational stress on symptoms of severe depression of the employees but there is no interaction found in this graph. It means that positive affectivity is not found as a significant moderator between the relationship of occupational stress and severe depression.

Chapter-VI

DISCUSSION

In this chapter, the obtained results have been discussed in the framework of relevant theoretical constructs and research literature relating to the problem of the present research.

With increasing importance of and attention towards positive psychological constructs or attributes at workplace, this study was conducted with the aim of examining the relationship between occupational stress and employees' physical and psychological health, and also analyze the buffering role of certain personal attributes on the adverse effect of occupational stress and health among supervisory level employees in public sector organizations. A moderate level of stress is actually necessary for survival. The stress reaction maximizes the expenditure of energy which helps prepare the body to meet the demands of a threatening or challenging situation and the individual tends to mobilize a great deal of effort in order to deal with the event. But beyond a certain level it affects individuals adversely and disrupt their physical, emotional, and psychological functioning, which lead to a variety of psychological and physical health problems. Present study in general revealed that physical as well as psychological heaths of the employees are adversely affected by the stress they experience at work. However, the positive personal attributes of the employees resist to occupational stress and significantly moderate the relationship between occupational stress and employee's health.

H1 proposed that "Occupational stress would be negatively correlated with health status".

As hypothesized the results of correlation analysis between occupational stress and ill-health and its dimensions indicate that occupational stress is positively related with ill-health and its four dimensions namely, somatic symptoms, anxiety/insomnia, social dysfunction and severe depression (Table 2). The reasons for high stress could be work overload because supervisors serves very pressure-filled job. In present study we found that supervisory level employees are experiencing high level of stress and as a result exhibit poor status of health. Similarly, the results of correlation analysis (Table 3) seems to suggest that all the dimensions of occupational stress, viz., role overload, role ambiguity, role conflict, unreasonable group and political pressures, under participation, powerlessness, poor peer relations, intrinsic impoverishment, low status, strenuous working conditions and unprofitability were significantly and positively associated with overall ill-health and its four dimensions.

However, stress arising from responsibility for persons, which is one of several dimensions of stress, was observed to be positively correlated, though insignificant by which suggest that responsibility for person was not a significant source of stress for supervisors. On the other hand, all other dimensions emerged out as strong stressors for employees. The results, taken as a whole, thus indicate that stress and health correlated significantly in the expected direction that is high stress associates with poor or ill-health and greater complaints of physical and psychological health problems by the supervisors.

In explanation of how occupational stress leads to health problem following facts may be extended. Though brain itself identifies threats, activities altering cognitive appraisals, coping processes, and integrates body reactions with filings, all parts of the body experience a major stress response. Following regions of the body system are particularly vulnerable to be affected by the experience of stress:

(a) Hypothalamic – pituitary – endocrine axis.
(b) Autonomic nervous system – adrenal medulla.
(c) Immune system.
(d) Reticular activating system.
(e) Involuntary and sustained muscle system.
(f) Cognitive – affective integrating system of the brain.

By engaging the integrating system, stress can cause health problems by:

(i) Lowering the immune response.
(ii) Creating endocrine problems through hyperactivity or hypoactivity.
(iii) Altering the balance of autonomic control, resulting in changes in cardio-vascular, respiratory, secretory and visceral system.
(iv) Altering sleep patterns with attendant impact on protein metabolism, hormone secretion, etc.
(v) Change in peptide release in extra CNS sites.
(vi) Affecting neurotransmitter, neuromodulator, and neuro-endocrine functions of brain.

The results of the present study have been found supporting the proposed first hypothesis, which are consistent with some earlier researches on daily hassles related stress, such as conflicts with family members or colleagues, work related problems, time pressure, conflict between job demands and financial difficulties, etc. Numerous studies have reported that occupational stress inversely related to psychological and physical health

(Banez & Compas, 1990; De Longis, Folkman, & Lazarus, 1988; Lai, 1995; Lai, Hamid, & Chow, 1996; De Jong et al., 1996). Stress has been noted to be associated with poor health of the individuals across the lifespan and in many cultures (Lin & Ensel, 1989; Marmot & Wilkinson, 1999).

Researchers estimated that stress plays an important role in 50 to 70% of all physical illnesses. Studies have also revealed that 60% of medical visits are primarily for stress related symptoms. Stress has also been linked to indicators of ill-health such as obesity, high systolic blood pressure, and elevated heart rates (Bell, Summerson, Spangler, & Konen, 2001; Brand, Hanson, & Godaert, 2000). A growing body of research suggests that stress is detrimental to mental and physical well-being (De Jong, timmerman, & Emmelkamp, 1996; Fabricatore et al., 2004).

A number of studies have reported that occupational stressors, such as heavy job demands and lack of control associate with various health problems. High-strain jobs have been linked with psychological distress, pain, and reduced physical functioning among nurses (Amick et al., 1998, Bourbonnais, Comeau, & Vezina, 1999), high demand or work-overload is the main cause of poor physical health (Carayon, 1993), increased job-tension/stress (Remontet & Hanssan, 1991), daily life stress (Carayon, 1993) and mental ill- health (Cooper & Kelly, 1993).

Researchers on stress have reported that stress at workplace arising from multiple role, role ambiguity, long working hours, overload, over commitment and responsibility of work and family was correlated with emotional exhaustion that leads to problems of depression, ulcer, neurotic symptoms, hypertension, frustration, depletion of energy, lowered resistance to illness, sickness absence, work errors and accident at work. Srivastava (1997) in his study noted that job-stress significantly associated with psychosomatic health complaints and pathological health habits. Sackeya and Sanda (2009) in their study noted that female managers experience greater work-related stress, which produce strain symptoms that function as predictors of their ill-health. The study by Fan, Blumenthal, Watkins, and Sherwood, (2015) revealed that work and home stress were significantly and strongly associated with anxiety and depression symptoms in both men and women.

H2 proposed that "Resilience would be positively correlated with health status"

The observed results (Table 2) indicate that resilience significantly and negatively correlates with overall ill-health and its four dimensions namely, somatic symptoms, anxiety/insomnia, social dysfunction and severe depression. On the basis of this finding we can say that when resilience increases the health of the supervisor also increases. If the supervisors are highly resilient the general heath of the supervisors would be high. Similarly, if the supervisors have low resilient personality, they would show poor symptoms of general health. It means that supervisors with high resilient attributes shows lower ill-health symptoms in stressful situations than lower resilient counterparts probably because the tendency of resilience protects the person from prolonged psychological and physiological reactions to adversities of life, which create risk for health strains and diseases for the persons.

Previous research findings suggest that resilience plays important role of a protective factor which protects the individual's psychological being and increases positive changes while coping with stressful situations (Dolbier, Jaggars, & Steinhardt, 2010; Kinman & Grant, 2011). Resilience seems to promote and maintain health and prevent illness (Muller, 2009).

Results of present study are in line with some other research findings. Mealer et al., (2012) found that high resilience associates with lesser symptoms of anxiety and depression. Anxiety and depression are one of the primary causes of ill-health in modern scenario due to high demands of work environment and social environment. Similarly, another study is also in support of present study (McGarry et al., 2014). He found that high resilience was associated with lower prevalence of burnout, symptoms of anxiety and depression among health professionals. His study clearly indicates that due to high resilient attitude/behavior there is low level of burnout, anxiety and depression in turns better health state.

Workplace stress has serious implications for the quality of an employee's work and their general psychological functioning. Researches investigating the relationship between psychological resilience and workforce related outcomes have consistently shown psychological resilience as to be inversely related to levels of psychological distress (Rees, Breen, Cusack & Hegney, 2015). Research findings mentioned above support our proposed second hypothesis.

H3 proposed that "Optimism would be positively correlated with health status"

The results of the correlational analysis between optimism and overall ill-health and its four dimensions (table 2) indicate that optimism negatively and significantly associated with overall ill-health status and its four dimensions namely, somatic symptoms, anxiety/insomnia, social dysfunction and severe depression. On the basis of the results it may be inferred that optimism plays a significant role in determining general health status of the supervisory personnel. It was noted that when optimism increases the health of supervisors also improved and they show lesser symptoms of ill-health. Similarly, if the supervisors have lower optimistic or pessimistic attributes, they will show more ill-health symptoms. Employees with optimistic attributes use more adaptive coping strategies. These types of employees are also likely to have the sense of control over their environment. The tendency of optimism and expectation of positive outcomes generate psychological strength in employee, which enhances his coping efficiency, general resistance and health status.

The findings of the present study are in conformity with earlier research on relationship between optimism and health. Optimism was found to be associated with better mental as well as physical health status (DeMoor et al., 2006). It has been noted that people with more optimistic and hopeful outlook are relatively less likely to become ill and also recover more quickly (Scheier et al., 2001). In a study it has been reported that individual having tendency of optimism have fewer illness complaints and are relatively at lower risk for premature mortality (Peterson & Seligman, 1987).

Optimism not only helps individuals in adapting to stressful events more successfully, but it also protects health (Taylor, Kemeny, Bower, Gruenewald, & Reed, 2000). It was shows in other studies that optimism plays a protective role against stress and depressive symptoms, and predicts higher health perceptions vitality and better mental health and lower bodily pain (Brissette et al., 2002; Achat et al., 2000). There is growing evidence that optimism is associated with better physical and mental health (Achat, Kawachi, Spiro, DeMolles, & Sparrow, 2000; Scheier & Carver, 1992; Segerstrom, Taylor, Kemeny, & Fahey, 1998).

It was reported that higher optimism is associated with fewer psychological symptoms (Plomin et al., 1992). Optimism was found to be strongly and positively related to psychological well-being and inversely related to distress among patients diagnosed with cancer (Miller, Manne, Taylor, Keates, & Dougherty, 1996). Optimism and expectancies for desirable outcomes have been positively associated with individual well-being in numerous studies (e.g., Aspinwall & Richter, 1999; Brissette, Scheier, & Carver, 2002; Scheier & Carver, 1985; Taylor, Lichtman, & Wood, 1984; Carver, Scheier, & Segerstrom, 2010).

Similarly positive effect of optimism has also been observed at the workplace. Tuten and Neidermeyer (2004) found that optimistic workers at call centers experienced lower level of job stress than their less optimistic peers; and Makikangas and Kinnunen (2003) also reported that optimism predicted lower mental distress among employees. These studies support our proposed third hypothesis that optimism would be positively correlated with health status. Optimism is a tendency to expect good things in the future. It is apparent that optimism is an attitude that heavily influences individual's coping with everyday stressors, and improve their physical as well as mental health.

H4 proposed that "Positive affectivity would be positively correlated with health status"

The results of the correlational analysis between positive affectivity and overall ill-health and its four dimensions namely, somatic symptoms, anxiety/insomnia, social dysfunction and severe depression observed (table 2) revealed that positive affectivity negatively but not significantly associates with overall ill-health and its dimensions except severe depression. Severe depression has been found to be negatively and significantly associated with positive affectivity. On the basis of this results findings it may be concluded that when positive affectivity increases general health of the supervisors also increases and they shows lower symptoms of ill-health. Similarly, on the other hand when positive affectivity is very low, the supervisor shows greater ill-health related symptoms. The result was not found to be significant, which means that positive affectivity has not play a significant role in determining health status of the supervisors.

The employees with high positive affectivity have a tendency to experience positive moods and emotions over time and across situation. Positive affectivity resists to illness and promotes health. This proposition has been supported by some previous studies. Positive emotion has been noted to increase people's physical, cognitive and social resources, which in turn help in effective coping and living healthier (Fredericson, 2001). People with high positive affectivity have longer life span, fewer pains and symptoms of illness (Cohen & Pressman, 2006).

Previous research findings established that individual high in positive affectivity view the world more in positive light and report leading full and interesting lives (Watson & Pennebaker, 1989). It was found that positive affect likely has a protective effect on health and also cited evidence that positive affect associates with lower morbidity, decreased symptoms and pain, and increased longevity (Pressman & Cohen, 2005).

Positive affect has been noted to enhance creative problem solving, which may help resolve stressful situations more quickly and consequently increase health protection (Ashby et al., 1999). Positive affectivity has found to be a good predictor of health and better prognosis form illness. Therefore, it is evident that positive affectivity is good for our health. Results were found supporting the proposed fourth hypothesis.

H5 proposed that "Resilience would moderate the relationship of occupational stress and health status"

The results (table 9) of the moderated regression analysis done to examine the moderating role of resilience on the relationship between occupational stress and ill-health (High score on the health scale indicates poor or ill-health) status, indicate that there has been gradual change in variance in decreasing order and this change is highly significant, which suggests that resilience emerged as a potential significant moderator of the relationship between stress and health. It moderated the adverse effect of stress on health of the supervisors. It is evident from figure 5.1 that, when resilience is low, the effect of occupational stress on health is higher and health became poor. However, when resilience is high, the effect of stress on health is reduced and the relationship between occupational stress and ill-health is weaker. Employees with high resilience show lower ill-health symptoms in stressful situations. In other words the employees have better health even in varying stressful situation than lower resilient counterparts.

The results of present study are in concordance with what was expected. The findings of the present study throw light on the extent to which employees engage in strategies to deal with stress and the success of those strategies depends largely upon characteristics of the employees. It is basically due to individual differences in cognitive appraisal and coping style that allow for the same stressor to be experienced by some as challenge and by others as hindrance. Those who are less resilient may turn to unhealthy actions or negative beliefs about themselves to cope with the difficulties encountered in their lives (Smokowski et al., 2000). According to Werner (2012) as well Noeker and Petermann (2008), resilient people are able to adapt to adverse, often traumatic environments, resulting in healthy long-term psychological functioning and better developmental outcomes.

Literature has gradually shifted focus to study resilience in the context of overcoming everyday moderate stress instead of chronic stresses like abuse and discrimination as it is also perceived as a stressor that may negatively impact an individual (DiCorcia & Tronick, 2011). It has been suggested that resilience buffers against the negative impacts of work stress, especially the inherently challenging working environments (Howard, 2008), positively coping with stressful events (Smokowski et al., 2000), or adaptive coping in the face of multiple risk factors (Waller et al., 2003).

It was found that resilience acts as a buffer which is likely to alleviate the impact of negative effect of job stress on the psychological health of supervisors (Kashyap, Kumar, & Krishna, 2014). Therefore, resilience acts as stress-resistant and implies the process where individuals are faced with acute or chronic stressors but are able to effectively maintain equilibrium under short-term significant strain. When individuals are exposed to prolonged or severe threat, and show a decrease in functioning, they are able to recover quicker than most when the threat is no longer present. Thus, resilience serves as a positive attribute of people to cope with stress.

H6 proposed that "Optimism would moderate the relationship of occupational stress and health status"

The results (table 14) of the moderated regression analysis done to examine the moderating role of optimism on the relationship between stress and ill-health (High score on the health scale indicates poor or ill-health), indicate that there has been gradual change in variance in decreasing order and this change is highly significant. The results suggest that optimism emerged as a potential significant moderator of the relationship between stress and health and it moderates the adverse effect of stress on health of the supervisors. From the interaction graph (Figure 5.6) it is evident that the positive relationship between occupational stress and ill-health is getting weaker when optimism is concerned. Results indicate that optimism buffers / moderates the negative impact of occupational stress on health by changing the direction of the relationship between these two.

From the graph it is evident that employees with high optimism show lesser poor health symptoms resulted from stressful situation. Optimists are more likely to view stressful work situations as challenging rather than threatening. As a characteristic of personality, optimism is assumed to protect the individual from the negative impacts of stress factors (Feldt, Mäkikangas, & Aunola, 2006; Mäkikangas et al., 2013).

Apart from supporting evidences of the results of the present study that optimism moderates the effects of stress on health status, some studies throw light on this. Dispositional optimism was found to significantly moderate the relation of stress and psychological well-being (Chang, 1998). Scheier and Carver (1992) found the moderating effect of optimism on the relationship between stressors and health.

It has been found that optimism exerts a moderating effect on the relationship between daily hassles and health outcomes (Fry, 1995), hassles and physiological symptoms (Lai, 1996), perceived stress and depression (Sumi, Horie, & Hayakawa, 1997), and psychosocial stressors and psychological well-being (Mäkikangas & Kinnunen, 2003).

H7 proposed that "Positive affectivity would moderate the relationship of occupational stress and health status"

The results (table 19) of moderated regression analyses, where in positive affectivity was taken as a moderator of the relationship between occupational stress and ill-health, indicate that the main effect of positive affectivity was not significant but interactional change has been found highly significant. This suggests that positive affectivity moderates the adverse effect of occupational stress on health. It can be said that in the present study positive affectivity emerged as a negative moderator of the relationship between stress and ill-health.

It is evident from the interaction graph of Figure 5.11 that under low stress condition, the different levels of positive affectivity do not aggravates the ill effects of occupational stress on health. However, under high occupational stress condition positive affectivity aggravates the ill effects of occupational stress on health of the employees. Hence we see that positive affectivity is a negative moderator of ill-health under high occupational stress condition.

The findings of the present study are in conformity with earlier research studies, which demonstrated that positive affect interacts with stress and moderates its negative effect on health (Davis et al., 2004; Faulk et al. 2012; Ong et al. 2006) such that the impact of stress on health is reduced when one's positive affect is high. It has been generally found that buffering functions of positive affectivity provide a useful antidote to the problem associated with negative emotions and ill-health caused from stress (Fredrickson, 2001).

Positive affect might influence appraisal of stressful situation and an individual's capacity to cope with stressors by promoting psychological resources, such as resilience and optimism. Positive affect promotes coping responses which lead to finding meaning in various stressful experiences (Khosla, 2006). It has also been noted that individuals who are better at coping with stress may handle stressful situations by activating or maintaining positive emotions (Tugade, Fredrickson, & Barrett, 2004) and having good health and well-being.

Study has also shown that happy individuals (i.e. those who experience positive affect) are successful in many areas, including job, marriage, and friendship (Lyubomirsky, King, & Diener, 2005). All these studies support our seventh hypothesis.

Therefore, in conclusion it can be said that individual's certain positive personal attributes play significant role in determining their health status and are the most important defense which people have against stress. It is important to build and foster positive attributes like, resilience, optimism, positive affectivity, etc. to be ready for future challenges, and to remain healthy which is important not only for employees of supervisory level but for all individuals as well.

CPSIA information can be obtained
at www.ICGtesting.com
Printed in the USA
LVHW081153241122
733912LV00015B/739

9 781805 450238